Sport Injury Prevention

ANATOMY

David Potach

Erik Meira

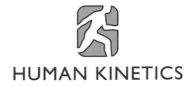

HUMAN KINETICS

Library of Congress Cataloging-in-Publication Data

Names: Potach, David, 1970- author. | Meira, Erik, 1976- author.
Title: Sport injury prevention anatomy / David Potach, Erik Meira.
Description: Champaign, IL : Human Kinetics, [2023] | Includes
  bibliographical references.
Identifiers: LCCN 2022002890 (print) | LCCN 2022002891 (ebook) | ISBN
  9781718208285 (print) | ISBN 9781718208292 (epub) | ISBN 9781718208308
  (pdf)
Subjects: LCSH: Sports injuries--Prevention. | Sports--Physiological
  aspects. | BISAC: HEALTH & FITNESS / Exercise / Stretching | MEDICAL /
  Sports Medicine
Classification: LCC RC1235 .P635 2023 (print) | LCC RC1235 (ebook) | DDC
  617.1/027--dc23/eng/20220318
LC record available at https://lccn.loc.gov/2022002890
LC ebook record available at https://lccn.loc.gov/2022002891

ISBN: 978-1-7182-0828-5 (print)

This publication is written and published to provide accurate and authoritative information relevant to the subject matter presented. It is published and sold with the understanding that the author and publisher are not engaged in rendering legal, medical, or other professional services by reason of their authorship or publication of this work. If medical or other expert assistance is required, the services of a competent professional person should be sought.

The web addresses cited in this text were current as of January 2022, unless otherwise noted.

Senior Acquisitions Editor: Michelle Earle; **Developmental Editor:** Amy Stahl; **Copyeditor:** Heather Gauen Hutches; **Permissions Manager:** Dalene Reeder; **Senior Graphic Designer:** Sean Roosevelt; **Cover Designer:** Keri Evans; **Cover Design Specialist:** Susan Rothermel Allen; **Illustrator (cover):** © Human Kinetics/Heidi Richter; **Photographs (for cover and interior illustration references):** © Human Kinetics/Jason Allen; **Photo Asset Manager:** Laura Fitch; **Photo Production Specialist:** Amy M. Rose; **Senior Art Manager:** Kelly Hendren; **Illustrations:** © Human Kinetics/Heidi Richter, Jen Gibas, and Jenn Tse; **Printer:** Versa Press

Human Kinetics books are available at special discounts for bulk purchase. Special editions or book excerpts can also be created to specification. For details, contact the Special Sales Manager at Human Kinetics.

Printed in the United States of America   10 9 8 7 6 5 4 3 2 1

The paper in this book is certified under a sustainable forestry program.

Human Kinetics
1607 N. Market Street
Champaign, IL 61820
USA

United States and International
Website: **US.HumanKinetics.com**
Email: info@hkusa.com
Phone: 1-800-747-4457

Canada
Website: **Canada.HumanKinetics.com**
Email: info@hkcanada.com

E8398

Tell us what you think!
Human Kinetics would love to hear what we can do to improve the customer experience. Use this QR code to take our brief survey.

Sport Injury Prevention

ANATOMY

CONTENTS

Introduction   vii

CHAPTER **1**   **UNDERSTANDING SPORT INJURIES**   **1**

CHAPTER **2**   **INJURY PREVENTION EXERCISE PRINCIPLES**   **9**

CHAPTER **3**   **HEAD, NECK, AND SHOULDER**   **21**

CHAPTER **4**   **ELBOW, WRIST, AND HAND**   **45**

CHAPTER **5**   **SPINE AND TRUNK**   **65**

CHAPTER **6**   **HIP**   **85**

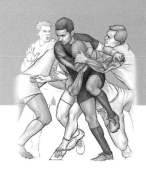

CHAPTER **7**   **THIGH**   **103**

CHAPTER **8**   **KNEE**   **129**

CHAPTER **9**   **LEG, ANKLE, AND FOOT**   **155**

CHAPTER **10**   **WARM-UP FOR INJURY PREVENTION**   **183**

CHAPTER **11**   **INJURY PREVENTION PROGRAM DESIGN**   **195**

Exercise Finder   205

References   208

About the Authors   219

Earn Continuing Education Credits/Units   222

INTRODUCTION

Being active is an important part of a lifelong healthy lifestyle. Physical activity improves heart and muscle health, boosts stamina and mental acuity, and helps control blood sugar and weight. Fortunately, many have gotten the message about the benefits of physical activity: Sport and exercise participation rates have generally increased over the past 20 years. Looking more deeply at these numbers, however, reveals that formal team sport participation rates have steadily decreased and that physical activity participation also decreases with age. Although reasons for these changes are multifactorial, one of the common causes is declining health and injury. Many athletes "retire" from sport participation at a young age because of injury and inability to return to their previous level of performance. Because of the many advantages of physical activity, it is beneficial to find ways to reduce the risk of injury and keep people actively involved in sport and exercise beyond their youth.

When applied to sport, exercise, and physical activity, the goal of injury prevention is to promote healthy lifestyles by reducing the risk of injury and improving the health and quality of life of both individual athletes and teams. This is best accomplished through the performance of specific exercises while following proper exercise or sport dosage and timing guidelines.

But is injury prevention possible? Before answering that question, it is important to appropriately define what is meant by *injury prevention*; this is more complex than it would first appear.

INJURY

An injury is defined as damage to a specific structure that often impairs intended function. Injuries are typically caused by the body's interaction with an external object—for example, a fall causes the body to contact the ground (external object) in such a way that injury may occur—but they can also occur as a result of acceleration, deceleration, changes of direction, playing too many games in too short of a period of time, or when the body is not properly prepared for games, activity, or exercise.

INJURY PREVENTION

The common use of the term *prevention* is to stop or keep something from happening, but it also means to slow, hinder, or forestall an event before it happens. Therefore, our definition of *injury prevention*—as discussed in the following chapters—is to reduce the likelihood of an injury occurring before it happens. We do not believe it is possible to stop all injuries from happening. Instead, we believe that proactively addressing specific risk factors before injuries occur—like performing certain exercises and using proper exercise and activity guidelines—can indeed prevent some injuries and reduce the risk and severity of others. We will continue using the term *prevention* but with the stated definition in mind.

DECREASED INJURY RATE

Whether targeting specific anatomical structures—like the ACL, ankle, or hamstring—or specific sports' athletes—like runners, wrestlers, or soccer players—the evidence is overwhelming that injury prevention programs do indeed reduce the risk of injury. In fact, some studies have shown that participation in these programs can decrease the risk of injury by up to 75 percent! Injury prevention programs that have been researched include those for specific injuries such as

- anterior cruciate ligament (ACL) tear (Ardern et al. 2018; Petushek et al. 2019; Tanaka et al. 2020),
- ankle sprain (Vuurberg et al. 2018),
- hamstring strain (Ayala et al. 2019; van Dyk et al. 2019),
- low back strain (Shiri et al. 2018),
- shoulder instability (Niederbracht et al. 2008), and
- concussion (Schneider et al. 2017).

This research also included injury prevention programs targeting specific sports and activities such as

- throwing (Wilk et al. 2021),
- running (Taddei et al. 2020; Warden et al. 2014),
- soccer (Crossley et al. 2020),
- wrestling (Grindstaff and Potach 2006),
- gymnastics (Sands 2000),
- dance (Fuller et al. 2020), and
- basketball (Cherni et al. 2019).

These programs—and more—have been shown to decrease injury risk. In addition, several organizations have published their own injury prevention programs. Most of these have focused on the ACL and include

- 11+ (formerly known as FIFA 11+) (FIFA Medical Network),
- Sportsmetrics (University of Cincinnati),
- PEP (Prevent injury, Enhance Performance) Program (Santa Monica Sports Medicine Research Foundation),

- Knäkontroll, and
- Thrower's Ten (American Sports Medicine Institute).

The general recommendation for all programs is to include various combinations of strength, plyometric, speed and agility, flexibility, and aerobic endurance exercises. Note, however, that flexibility exercises for injury prevention have shown mixed results.

INJURY PREVALENCE

Participation in injury prevention programs is recommended for all athletes but is especially important for those athletes in sports that require frequent landings, deceleration, and changes of direction, such as soccer, basketball, football, and volleyball; athletes in these sports tend to get injured at higher rates than those in other sports. Injury prevention is also recommended for baseball players, who are at an increased risk of shoulder and elbow injury—especially pitchers and catchers, whose positions involve a higher total number of throws as well as throws at high velocities.

Although males account for the highest overall number of ACL injuries, females in sports like soccer and basketball have up to six times greater risk of injury than their male counterparts—an injury rate similar to male football players. Because of these rates, we recommend all female athletes—especially those playing sports in high-risk categories, like soccer and basketball—and male football players be specifically targeted to participate in ACL injury prevention programs.

PARTICIPATION

Unfortunately, although nearly 90 percent of athletes expressed interest in participating in an injury prevention program when asked (Martinez et al 2017), fewer than 20 percent have performed such programs. Furthermore, fewer than 33 percent of youth soccer coaches have their athletes perform injury prevention programs. Some of the proposed barriers to this participation include the following:

- *Lack of education.* However, when educated, only half of coaches had their athletes perform exercises (Sugimoto et al 2017).
- *Lack of awareness.* Only 33 percent of athletes are aware that such programs exist (Tanaka 2020).
- *Lack of time.* Though most programs take less than 15 minutes to perform, many coaches are unwilling to sacrifice practice time for this purpose.

The goal of this text is to give you a basic understanding of why injuries occur, the principles behind injury prevention programs, and common injury prevention exercises you can perform to reduce injury risk. Although designing and performing these exercise programs will not guarantee you won't get hurt, we believe that with a small investment of time, your risk of injury will significantly decrease and, as an added benefit, your performance should likewise improve.

To do this, we will provide general physiological and training principles used to design injury prevention programs. This background material will be followed by chapters that include detailed descriptions of exercises that reduce the risk of specific injuries. These exercises will include the exercise mode, steps for performing the exercise, the muscles involved, and a Preventive Focus section to highlight what injury the exercise is best for preventing. In each exercise in the subsequent chapters, you will see three icons, one for each of the three exercise modes: strength training exercises, plyometric exercises, and special training exercises, respectively (see icons). The purpose of these icons is to identify the exercise mode or modes that predominantly apply to the exercise; the applicable mode will be shown in full-color versus the screened-back icons that do not apply to the exercise. These three exercise modes are described in full detail in chapter 2.

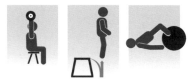

To help guide you, each exercise will be accompanied by an anatomical illustration that demonstrates how each exercise is performed. Due to the positioning of the exercises, you may not be able to see all the involved muscles in the exercise illustrations; all of the muscles involved are listed in a separate section within each exercise. Some exercise illustrations will have instances where a muscle is only easily visible on a nonworking extremity; in those instances you will see the labels appear on those visible nonworking extremities instead of the working extremities in the exercise. In addition, these illustrations are color coded to indicate the primary and secondary muscles and the connective tissues featured in each exercise.

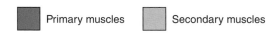

The book will conclude with a chapter that combines the physiological and training principles with specific exercises to guide you through the process of designing an injury prevention program. This chapter will include an example of an injury prevention program.

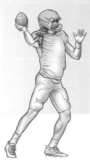

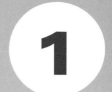

UNDERSTANDING SPORT INJURIES

Injury prevention requires the thoughtful use of specific exercises, appropriate intensity, proper technique, and sound training practices. If just one of these factors is ignored, effectiveness can be compromised. This book will identify specific injuries and how they typically occur, as well as provide exercises that directly address those injuries. However, an understanding of injury basics is important to effectively use the strategies that will be covered in later chapters. While this book is about reducing the risk of sport related injuries, many of the principles apply to other activities, including those related to exercise, fitness, and even work.

Injury is relatively easy to understand. An injury is, quite simply, damage to a specific structure that often impairs intended function. There are four parts to this definition:

1. *Damage* indicates that the integrity of the structure has changed (e.g., a break or rupture).
2. *Specific structure* refers to the anatomy involved (e.g., a bone or tendon).
3. *Impairs* means that the structure can no longer fully perform its job (e.g., decreased joint stability or force production).
4. *Function* is a specific goal-oriented task (e.g., running or climbing stairs).

A common injury for soccer players is a hip flexor strain. When shooting a soccer ball on goal, the hip flexor muscle fibers (most commonly those of rectus femoris) can tear either partially or completely. This muscle fiber tearing is the definition of a *strain*. When strained, the rectus femoris can often still perform its task of flexing the thigh at the hip, but it causes pain, which commonly decreases the force that the rectus femoris is able to produce, resulting in decreased velocity when shooting the ball. Referring to our definition of *injury*, a strain (or tearing of muscle fibers) is the damage, the rectus femoris muscle is the specific structure, decreased force production is the impairment, and the effectiveness of shooting a soccer ball is the function.

One way to define or classify injuries is based on both the structure involved and the mechanism that caused the injury. Some injuries, termed *traumatic*, are the result of a specific episode, whereas other injuries, termed *overuse*, occur over time. Both types of injury occur because the involved tissues—like muscles, ligaments, tendons, and bones—are unable to tolerate the stresses experienced. Stress is not necessarily a problem unless the stress applied is greater than the structure's maximal tolerance. For example, performing a typical repetition of the bench press stresses the muscles involved with the movement (specifically pectoralis major, anterior deltoid, and triceps brachii), but for most people, this stress is well tolerated and no injury occurs. But what might happen if a novice lifter attempts to perform a one-repetition maximum (1RM) for his first lift? Or if an experienced lifter doubles the volume of her usual routine? In the first example, if the force required of the untrained pectoralis major is greater than the amount of force that it can withstand, a traumatic injury can occur. In the second example, if the force experienced over a period of time is greater than the pectoralis major has been trained to encounter, an overuse injury can occur.

TRAUMATIC INJURIES

Traumatic injuries occur when a single episode of stress—or force—introduced to a body structure exceeds its tolerance. Sometimes these forces are introduced externally (as with contact with an object or opposing player), and sometimes they are introduced internally (as with a muscle). Most anatomical structures can be traumatically injured. The following are some common traumatic injuries:

- Ankle sprains involve the tearing of lateral (outside) ligament fibers and commonly occur when the foot turns inward (inversion) to a degree greater than the ligaments can tolerate.
- Achilles tendon ruptures—tearing of the fibers connecting the main lower leg plantar flexors to the heel—occur when greater forces are transmitted through the tendon than it can tolerate.
- Radius bone fractures can occur when an athlete falls onto an outstretched hand, transmitting a force greater than the bone can tolerate.
- Shoulder dislocations or subluxations often occur when an athlete's shoulder moves too far anteriorly, introducing a force greater than the glenohumeral labrum—a stabilizing rim of cartilage in the shoulder—can tolerate.
- Traumatic injuries to the hamstring muscle group commonly occur while it is producing a high amount of force and is then required to produce more force than it can tolerate (due to position, speed, or both).

The common thread to all of those types of injuries is a structure experiencing a greater force than it can tolerate during a specific episode. Traumatic injuries can be further classified as direct contact, indirect contact, or noncontact injuries. Classifying traumatic injuries in this manner refers to the environment in which the injury occurs and how force develops in the system.

Direct Contact Injury

A direct contact injury occurs when a structure sustains a direct blow. For example, if a football player falls into a kneeling position and another player lands on his ankle, twisting the lower leg against a fixed knee, it can result in a direct contact high ankle sprain. This injury results from a different mechanism and involves different ligaments than a typical inversion ankle sprain. Another common direct contact injury is a fractured bone—for example, if a person is weight training and drops a weight plate on her foot, the result may be a fractured bone.

Indirect Contact Injury

In contrast to a direct contact injury, an indirect contact injury occurs when there is contact with another player, but not directly to the involved structure. For example, if an athlete's right knee is hit directly by an opponent, resulting in injury, that is a direct contact injury. But, if the athlete is hit by an opponent at the shoulder, resulting in a right knee injury as the athlete braces against that contact, that is an indirect contact injury.

There are two common indirect contact situations that can result in injuries:

- When an athlete is injured because of their reaction to contact with another player
- When an athlete is pushed while in the air and an injury results upon landing

Noncontact Injury

Noncontact injuries occur—as the name suggests—when no part of the athlete is touching a different object or player. For example, when a football player is running at high speed, changes direction, and inverts his ankle, this is a noncontact ankle sprain. Though less common than contact-related fractures, noncontact bone fractures may also occur; for example, a basketball player landing from a rebound may fracture a bone in the lower leg.

Anterior Cruciate Ligament Injury

The anterior cruciate ligament (ACL) lies in front of (anterior) and crosses (cruciate) the posterior cruciate ligament (PCL). The three contact classifications can all result in an ACL tear:

- *Direct contact.* Another athlete collides directly with the knee, forcing it into a direction that tears the ACL.
- *Indirect contact.* Another athlete collides with the player, resulting in a tear of the ACL as the player braces against that contact.
- *Noncontact.* A player is decelerating or changing direction and an inward (valgus) movement and a lack of flexion of the knee results in a tear of the ACL.

Although a noncontact injury technically occurs with no physical contact from another athlete, that does not mean that there are no outside forces contributing to the injury. Often, the injury is a result of the athlete's quick reactions to unique situations. For example, a rugby player may start to accelerate in one direction only to realize that an opposing player is there, and the attempt to quickly redirect may result in a tear of the ACL. It could be said that the interaction with the other player resulted in an injury, even though no physical contact was made. This is more complicated than "moving wrong" in general.

OVERUSE INJURIES

Although traumatic injuries result from the body experiencing too much stress during a single instant, overuse injuries occur when body structures encounter stress they cannot tolerate over a prolonged period without adequate recovery.

Ligaments

Consider pitching a baseball. Baseball pitchers are typically called upon to throw dozens of high-speed pitches in a relatively short period of time. To throw at a high speed, great forces are initiated by the muscles and surrounding tissues of both the upper and lower body, particularly those surrounding the shoulder and elbow joints. If performed one time, or if spread out over a longer period with adequate rest, injury is not as likely to occur, but pitchers usually pitch dozens of times in a single game, with only 15 to 20 minutes of rest between innings. This can lead to overuse injuries of several structures, like the ulnar collateral ligament (UCL), the ligament involved in the increasingly common Tommy John surgical procedure. Combine the high forces, large volume of pitches, and relatively short rest and recovery, and overuse injury is likely to occur.

Bones

Running is another activity prone to cause overuse injury. On average, runners take up to 200 steps per minute; over a 30-minute run, that is 6,000 steps. If the runner averages four days per week, that is 24,000 steps. Because several muscles are involved with both the push-off and landing of the running cycle, increased stress is introduced to those tissues as well as those adjacent to them. In this case, the tissues adjacent to them are bones; in other words, this combination of step volume, impact, and repeated pull of the muscles on the bones can lead to shin splints or bone stress reactions—or even stress fractures—of the tibia.

Tendons

Playing basketball is another activity that can result in overuse injury. The most common overuse injury for this athlete is the so-called "jumper's knee," a tendinopathy of the patellar tendon (the structure that connects the large quadriceps muscles to the lower leg through the kneecap). These muscles help the athlete to jump, but also help control landing and deceleration. With rebounds, jump shots, and quick changes of direction, basketball involves a lot of these motions, and this heavy volume of loading cycles can contribute to an overloading of the patellar tendon, resulting in a tendinopathy.

FACTORS THAT CONTRIBUTE TO INJURY RISK

The goal of this text is to reduce the risk of injury. To do this, it is important to review the reasons injuries occur in the first place. Once those are known, programs can be designed to address those reasons, thereby reducing the risk of injury. Understanding how injuries occur requires a thoughtful analysis of forces encountered by athletes in various sports, how those forces are tolerated, and techniques that are commonly associated with injury. Aside from those common causes, other variables can contribute to injury, such as progressing a program too quickly (or too slowly), the athlete's previous experience in sport, and even athlete fitness. We will cover each of these and will describe how they can affect an athlete's risk of injury.

Force

Force is simply the effect of one body on another, like the push or a pull applied to an object to attempt to change its state of motion. In the human body, this force is an interaction between internal and external resistance to movement—internal forces are initiated from *within* the body to change motion, whereas external forces are initiated from *outside* the body due to its interaction with the surrounding environment.

Force is always an interaction between two or more objects, so there cannot be an internal force without an equal and opposite external force. For simplicity, we will often describe them in isolation, such as "muscle force," even though in reality it is always an interaction.

Although internal forces can be a reaction such as compression, the most common internal forces are tensile muscle forces, which are generated to pull on bones to create motion. One other type of internal force is joint reaction force, which describes the forces generated by bone-on-bone contact between adjacent body segments. These joint reaction forces represent the net effects that are transmitted from one segment to another and are due to the muscle, ligament, and bony contact forces exerted across a joint. Think of the knees of a basketball player landing from a jump: When his feet hit the ground, the interaction with the ground results in force being applied to the athlete's body. As his knees bend to absorb those forces, the quadriceps muscles resist that bending in order to control the landing. The interaction of the flexion impulse from the landing and the extension impulse from the quadriceps results in a joint reaction force.

External forces involve contact between the athlete and something outside of—external to—the athlete's body, most commonly as a result of gravity or contact with another object or person. For example, blocking or tackling an opponent results in one person contacting another; pushing off the wall when swimming involves the swimmer contacting and transmitting force to the wall; and landing from a jump causes contact between the athlete's feet and the ground.

When any of these forces exceed the tolerance of the structures encountering them, injury can occur, for example:

- Excess tensile forces in the muscle can result in muscle strain
- Excess joint reaction force can result in cartilage damage
- Excess shear force can result in skin abrasion

Technique

Technique refers to the organization—and ultimately the execution—of a given movement. Although there is no specific right or wrong way to perform a given movement, some techniques are more commonly associated with injuries because the body can often tolerate certain techniques better than others.

- Excessive valgus (inward) movement is associated with ACL tear.
- Landing toward the front of the foot when running can result in increased stress at the ankle joint.
- Throwing from a sidearm position can result in increased stress to the medial (inside) part of the elbow.

Using these techniques does not necessarily mean injury will occur. Rather, these techniques are merely associated with increased occurrence of injuries.

Training Stress

The body can respond to training stresses in a number of ways. When training, progression of stresses—most commonly prescribed by manipulating training variables like volume, intensity, frequency, and duration—must occur for the desired progression of adaptations to occur, such as improved performance. If no progression of stresses occurs—or if progression is at too low a level—then little to no improvement will occur. If the training stresses are progressed too quickly, injury becomes more likely. When and how much to progress should change based on both the athlete's ability and the time of year (e.g., in-season or offseason). When evaluating injury risk, then, it is important to consider both the exercises performed as well as the progress of the identified training stresses.

Fitness Level

Research has yet to determine an ideal level of fitness for sporting participation. There is no magic strength, flexibility, power, or aerobic level considered a prerequisite to sport involvement. However, it has been our experience—and research tends to suggest this as well—that the more "in shape" an athlete is, the less likely she is to become injured. This is not necessarily the same across all sports—some sports favor flexibility, others favor power, whereas still others benefit most from strength. The closer to ideal each of these variables is, the less likely an athlete is to become injured.

Sport Experience

A final factor to consider is how much experience an athlete has. Human movement solutions are acquired through complex learning mechanisms in extremely specific environments. This is most naturally accomplished through the athletes' experiences playing their sport. In other words, as athletes spend more time playing their sport, they collect more experience not just with the sport in general, but with the unique situations that can develop during competition.

Think about the previous example of an injury that occurs when an athlete reacts to the sudden appearance of an opposing player blocking his intended direction of movement. If this is a situation that the athlete has been in many times before, he will have ample experience to draw upon to form an ideal response. If the athlete has not encountered this situation many times before, then he may not know how to effectively and safely react to avoid contact with the blocking player and therefore avoid possible injury. This increased sport experience and exposure can build tolerance to activity, resulting in an increased resilience to injury. Proper injury prevention programming therefore must include frequent participation in the activity.

The chapters that follow will provide you with exercises and strategies to reduce some of the most common injuries athletes experience. Some injuries simply cannot be avoided, but by building a more resilient athlete, we can greatly reduce their risk of injury. Most athletes will benefit from the proper application of force and training stresses to optimize training outcomes.

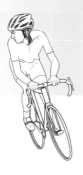

2

INJURY PREVENTION EXERCISE PRINCIPLES

When designing an injury prevention program, several variables must be addressed to ensure that participants are safe and the program is effective. A great deal of time and understanding is required to properly incorporate an injury prevention program into an overall training plan. Injury types and exercise principles are essential to designing a program for athletes; using and adhering to those principles maximizes the chances of the athlete's success while also reducing the likelihood of injury. An overview of the various types of injuries were covered in the previous chapter, and now we will discuss the principles of exercise design. The exercise principles that we focus on in this book include types of muscle contractions, selection of exercise types, and how humans learn movement.

Specificity, overload, and progression are perhaps the most important considerations when choosing exercises to include in an injury prevention program. We must consider how the body moves and how the muscles function during both general movement and the specific moments during which the body is most susceptible to injury. If the loads do not challenge the athlete—i.e., overload—adaptations will not occur. And if the exercises and loads are not progressed through exercise complexity or weight, the athlete will plateau and continued adaptations will suffer. Therefore, when designing injury prevention programs, our goal is to bring about certain changes or adaptations specific to the type of demand imposed upon the body. This is referred to as *specific adaptation to imposed demands,* or the *SAID principle.* If the goal is to run faster, fast running should be included in the training program; if the goal is to jump higher, jumping should be included in the training program.

MOVEMENT DESCRIPTION

To analyze sport movements and use exercises to help reduce injury risk, an understanding of movement terminology is important. All sporting function involves the coordinated movement of the body's joints. This movement is purposely controlled by muscle contractions. As those contractions move the joints and encounter resistance to that movement, force is generated, called *torque*. The most common joint movements are provided in figure 2.1.

Wrist—sagittal
Flexion
Exercise: wrist curl
Sport: basketball free throw

Extension
Exercise: wrist extension
Sport: racquetball backhand

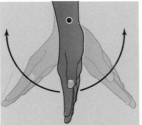

Wrist—frontal
Ulnar deviation
Exercise: ulnar deviation wrist curl
Sport: baseball bat swing

Radial deviation
Exercise: radial deviation wrist curl
Sport: golf backswing

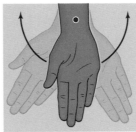

Elbow—sagittal
Flexion
Exercise: biceps curl
Sport: bowling

Extension
Exercise: triceps pushdown
Sport: shot put

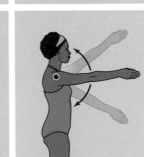

Shoulder—sagittal
Flexion
Exercise: front shoulder raise
Sport: boxing uppercut punch

Extension
Exercise: neutral-grip seated row
Sport: freestyle swimming stroke

Shoulder—frontal
Adduction
Exercise: wide-grip lat pulldown
Sport: swimming breast stroke

Abduction
Exercise: wide-grip shoulder press
Sport: springboard diving

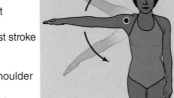
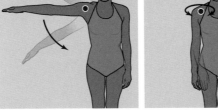

Shoulder—transverse or horizont
Internal rotation
Exercise: internal rotation with tubing
Sport: baseball pitch

External rotation
Exercise: external rotation with tubin
Sport: martial arts movement

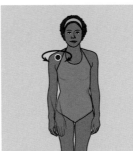

FIGURE 2.1 Common joint movements used in sport.
Adapted by permission from E.A. Harman, M. Johnson, and P.N. Frykman, "A Movement-Oriented Approach to Exercise Prescription," *NSCA Journal* 14, no. 1 (1992): 47-54.

Shoulder—transverse or horizontal
(upper arm to 90° to trunk)
Adduction
Exercise: dumbbell chest fly
Sport: tennis forehand

Abduction
Exercise: bent-over lateral raise
Sport: tennis backhand

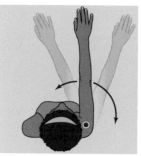

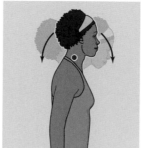

Neck—sagittal
Flexion
Exercise: neck machine
Sport: somersault

Extension
Exercise: dynamic back bridge
Sport: back tuck

Neck—transverse or horizontal
Left rotation
Exercise: manual resistance
Sport: wrestling movement

Right rotation
Exercise: manual resistance
Sport: wrestling movement

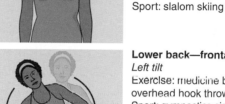

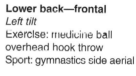
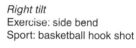

Neck—frontal
Left tilt
Exercise: neck machine
Sport: slalom skiing

Right tilt
Exercise: neck machine
Sport: slalom skiing

Lower back—sagittal
Flexion
Exercise: sit-up
Sport: javelin throw follow-through

Extension
Exercise: hyperextension
Sport: back tuck

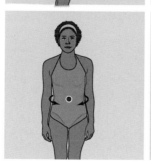

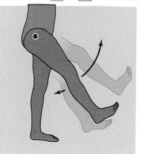

Lower back—frontal
Left tilt
Exercise: medicine ball overhead hook throw
Sport: gymnastics side aerial

Right tilt
Exercise: side bend
Sport: basketball hook shot

Lower back—transverse or horizontal
Left rotation
Exercise: medicine ball side toss
Sport: baseball batting

Right rotation
Exercise: torso machine
Sport: golf swing

Hip—sagittal
Flexion
Exercise: leg raise
Sport: American football punt

Extension
Exercise: back squat
Sport: long jump take-off

(continued)

FIGURE 2.1   *(continued)*

Hip—frontal
Adduction
Exercise: standing adduction machine
Sport: soccer side step

Abduction
Exercise: standing abduction machine
Sport: hockey skating

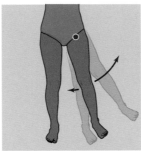

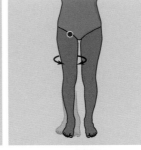

Hip—transverse
Internal rotation
Exercise: resisted internal rotation
Sport: basketball pivot movement

External rotation
Exercise: resisted external rotation
Sport: figure skating turn

Hip—transverse or horizontal
(upper leg to 90° to trunk)
Adduction
Exercise: adduction machine
Sport: karate in-sweep

Abduction
Exercise: seated abduction machine
Sport: wrestling escape

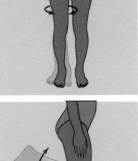

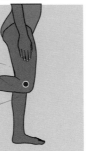

Knee—sagittal
Flexion
Exercise: stability ball hamstring curl
Sport: diving tuck

Extension
Exercise: leg extension
Sport: volleyball block

Ankle—sagittal
Dorsiflexion
Exercise: resisted ankle dorsiflexion
Sport: running

Plantar flexion
Exercise: calf (heel) raise
Sport: high jump

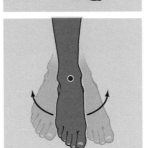

Ankle—frontal
Inversion
Exercise: resisted inversion
Sport: change of direction in soccer

Eversion
Exercise: resisted eversion
Sport: speed skating

FIGURE 2.1   *(continued)*

Adapted by permission from E.A. Harman, M. Johnson, and P.N. Frykman, "A Movement-Oriented Approach to Exercise Prescription," *NSCA Journal* 14, no. 1 (1992): 47-54.

MUSCLES AND MOVEMENT

In order to describe the relationship between muscles and movement, we will examine three separate but related purposes. Specifically, we consider the muscle's function, the muscle's action, and the speed of the muscle contraction.

Muscle Function

A muscle's function is a description of how it engages in response to external stimulus. (*Note*: Although there is a slight difference between a muscle's function and role, the two terms are used interchangeably here.) There are two components to determining muscle function: force generation and movement. When a muscle contracts, it generates force. Sometimes this force produces movement (e.g., jumping up), sometimes it resists movement (e.g., decelerating when landing), and sometimes it maintains position (e.g., iron cross movement in gymnastics). Generating force and the associated type of movement is referred to as *muscle contraction* or *action*, but both muscle force and type of movement are important to this definition. If a partner bends an athlete's elbow but the athlete does not assist, this is not a muscle action, it is a passive movement. Although there is some debate about using the term *muscle contraction* (contraction refers to shortening) versus *muscle action*, we will use the term *muscle contraction* here for ease of reading and understanding.

Muscles have different roles—to produce or resist movement—based on the movement's goal. The three roles we will discuss are agonist, antagonist, and stabilizer. An agonist is the prime mover of a given action. For a dumbbell biceps curl, the muscles of the arm (primarily brachialis and biceps brachii) are the agonists—the muscles generating the force to produce the movement. Antagonist muscles oppose the given movement. In the case of the dumbbell biceps curl, triceps brachii is the antagonist muscle group. Stabilizers help maintain body alignment to perform the movement. During the dumbbell biceps curl, the shoulder muscles (primarily deltoid and the rotator cuff muscles) maintain shoulder alignment to allow the movement at the elbow.

Muscle Action

A muscle action is the description of what happens when a muscle contracts. As mentioned, all muscle contractions result in the generation of force. There are three primary types of muscle contractions that refer to the type of movement that results from that generation of force: concentric, eccentric, and isometric.

Concentric

Concentric muscle contractions refer to those muscle actions that involve shortening of the muscle. During concentric contractions, the muscle fibers shorten and bring the ends of the fibers closer together. The result of this concentric action is movement at the joint. It is easiest to think of concentric muscle contractions as *producing* movement. When performing the upward phase of the dumbbell biceps curl, the anterior muscles of the arm (primarily brachialis and biceps brachii) are concentrically active to bend the elbow and therefore raise the weight. In this scenario, the arm muscles generate more internal force than the external force produced by the external resistance of the dumbbell, and the dumbbell is lifted. Cycling is an example of an activity that is almost entirely concentric in nature.

Eccentric

Eccentric muscle contractions refer to those muscle actions that involve lengthening of the muscle. During eccentric contractions, the muscle fibers get longer, and the ends of the fibers move farther apart. It is easiest to think of eccentric muscle contractions as resisting movement. When performing the downward phase of the dumbbell biceps curl, the same anterior muscles of the arm are now eccentrically active to resist extension of the elbow and therefore lower the weight slowly. In this scenario, the arm muscles generate less internal force than the external force produced by the resistance of the dumbbell, and the dumbbell is lowered. Landing from a jump is an example of an activity that is almost entirely eccentric in nature. Throwing a baseball or softball also requires eccentric muscle action. Once the ball has been released, the muscles on the posterior aspect of the shoulder (infraspinatus, teres minor, posterior deltoid, rhomboids) act eccentrically to slow down the momentum of the arm.

Two primary benefits of exercises involving eccentric contractions are the ability to improve tolerance to eccentric exercise—a sort of "injury proofing" of the muscles—and the role eccentric contractions play in deceleration. First, when eccentric exercises are performed, a phenomenon referred to as *delayed onset muscle soreness* (DOMS) often occurs. DOMS involves the microtearing of muscle fibers, which causes swelling and pain 48 hours after exercise. Continuing to perform exercises with an eccentric bias is a strategy to improve tolerance to that motion or activity. Running downhill is a good example: The quadriceps contract eccentrically to function as brakes for the body to slow down the descent, often causing significant soreness in the front of a runners' thighs. But if done repeatedly, tolerance to this muscle contraction increases and the likelihood of future soreness eventually decreases.

In addition, muscles act in an eccentric fashion when decelerating motion. Most sports involve repeated bouts of stopping, starting, slowing down, and changing direction. This period of stopping and changing direction is a common moment of injury. During those stops and changes of direction, the involved muscles act eccentrically to slow or stop the athlete's motion, or momentum, before acting concentrically to begin moving again. Because momentum is the product of mass and velocity, both larger and faster objects require greater force to slow or stop. If we are able to train the muscles to more efficiently decelerate the body—via eccentric muscle action—we can decrease the risk of injury.

Isometric

Isometric muscle contractions refer to those actions that involve the muscle essentially remaining the same length. During isometric contractions, the muscle fibers remain active, but the ends of the fibers remain the same distance apart. It is easiest to think of isometric muscle contractions as *maintaining* position. For example, if the athlete pauses during one of the phases of the dumbbell biceps curl and holds the dumbbell in place without moving, the muscles of the anterior arm are isometrically active to maintain position of the elbow. In this scenario, the arm muscles generate the same internal force as the external force produced by the resistance of the dumbbell, and the dumbbell is stationary. Holding a plank position is an example of an activity that is almost entirely isometric in nature.

Speed of Contraction

Muscle contractions can be slow and controlled, but they also occur during rapid movements. The speed of muscle contraction that occurs during an athlete's sport is important to consider when designing injury prevention exercises. For example, throwing a ball involves several phases, generally summarized as rapid agonist eccentric muscle contraction, followed by rapid agonist concentric contraction, and ending with rapid antagonist eccentric contraction. When training to reduce throwing-related injuries, exercises should be included that consider these rapid movements; if only slow exercises are provided for a thrower, strength will increase, but it will not be specific to the type of muscle contraction required by the athlete.

Special thought must be given to exercises that focus on power production. As opposed to the three primary types of muscle contractions, during which athletes commonly use slow or controlled movements, explosive contractions involve the athlete moving with maximum concentric acceleration. Although this maximum speed of muscle contraction can occur from a resting position, it is often preceded by an eccentric contraction. Furthermore, these explosive muscle contractions can occur when no movement takes place.

However, it is easiest to think of explosive muscle contractions as accelerating rapidly. If the athlete performs the dumbbell biceps curl by lifting the dumbbell as quickly and forcefully as possible, this would be an explosive muscle contraction: The anterior arm muscles rapidly generate more internal force than the external force produced by the resistance of the dumbbell, creating a swift momentum change. However, the dumbbell biceps curl exercise is not a common use of explosive muscle contractions, which are more commonly seen during jumping, cutting, and throwing. These activities involve the rapid generation of force to produce—and resist—large and quick changes of momentum.

Motor Learning

Learning to perform a movement task is a complex process of trial and error between the athlete and the surrounding physical world. This process is commonly referred to as *motor learning*. Within the athlete is a complicated interface between the nervous system and the musculoskeletal system, with a near-infinite number of possible nuanced solutions. Therefore, the optimal solution for a movement task for one athlete might be different from the optimal solution for another.

The ideal training strategy may be to manipulate the environment to encourage each athlete to explore and find their own best solution. Understanding basic biomechanical principles, exercise modes, and activity exposure is key to developing the ideal training environment for each unique athlete.

BIOMECHANICAL PRINCIPLES

Injury prevention program design relies on the many principles of biomechanics to be effective. When analyzing athletic movements, we most often focus on how force is applied. Sometimes it is applied quickly to produce motion (rate of force development), sometimes it is held for a long period (strength endurance), and sometimes it is needed to slow down movement (deceleration). The easiest way to think of these applications is to consider the force that is produced over time when pushing against a fixed object and the resulting force–time curve (impulse; see figure 2.2).

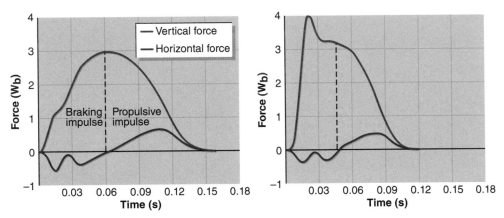

FIGURE 2.2   Force–time curve.

Reprinted by permission from B.H. Deweese and S. Nimphius, "Program Design and Technique for Speed and Agility Training," in *Essentials of Strength Training and Conditioning,* 4th ed., edited for the National Strength and Conditioning Association by G.G. Haff and N.T. Triplett (Champaign, IL: Human Kinetics, 2016), 524.

Force

Force is the push or pull on an object by another object. This tends to result in a change in the state of rest or motion of that object—in other words, force creates a change of momentum. The body experiences many types of force. Some are internal, like the pulling of a muscle or the stiffness of a bone, and some are external, like the friction of a running surface or the impact of hitting the ground. Peak force is represented by the highest point achieved on the force–time curve.

Rate of Force Development

Rate of force development (RFD) refers to how quickly force is generated. This is represented by the slope at any given point of the force–time curve. RFD can be looked at two different ways. It is an indicator of an athlete's explosive strength; greater RFD results in more explosiveness. Another way to view RFD is by looking at how much stress an athlete can tolerate. Specifically, the more quickly that an athlete can generate internal force via muscle contraction, the higher amounts of quickly developing external forces that the athlete can tolerate.

Impulse

Impulse is force produced over time and is represented by the area under the force–time curve. The amount of impulse that can be generated in a given time limits the amount of momentum that can change in the same amount of time. In sporting actions such as landing and cutting, there is a very short amount of time available to generate impulse. If the athlete can generate a high peak force, but not in the available window of time, the resulting change in momentum will not be as great as desired. Impulse, then, is a combination of the proper amount of force applied for the proper amount of time.

Strength Endurance

The ability to produce a given amount of force over a prolonged period is known as *strength endurance*. In sport and exercise, athletes are often required to maintain a position for a long period of time, like holding a plank or performing the iron cross in gymnastics. Variations of strength endurance include speed endurance (e.g., maintaining running speed over a prolonged time, like a middle-distance runner) and explosive endurance (e.g., producing repeated explosive contractions over a prolonged time, like a basketball center rebounding).

Deceleration

As described earlier, deceleration is the process of rapidly slowing the body. Deceleration is most often seen in sports that require an immediate or gradual stop or frequent changes in direction. Deceleration requires significant eccentric muscle contractions, typically over a very short period of time, to help with this rapid change of momentum.

EXERCISE MODES

Program design can involve several types—or modes—of exercise. There are multiple ways to categorize these modes of exercise; however, we will focus on five modes: strength, plyometric, speed and agility, flexibility, and aerobic endurance training. In the introduction, you will find details on the icons that will appear with each exercise to indicate the exercise mode.

Strength Training

Strength training—often used interchangeably with resistance training, weight training, or weightlifting—is the use of resistance to increase strength in specific muscles. Sometimes this resistance is simply gravity, as with bodyweight exercises; sometimes this resistance may be an external weight like a dumbbell or barbell. The dumbbell overhead shoulder press and the bodyweight squat are two common strength training exercises.

Strength training exercises are typically performed using slow, controlled movements, but certain strength training exercises allow athletes to target specific goals, like power. One example is the power clean, which involves lifting a barbell from the floor to the shoulders in a rapid, powerful manner. Strength training is the foundation of most injury prevention programs because this training is relatively easy to do and it is supported by several research studies.

Plyometric Training

Plyometric training is the use of exercises to produce maximal force in the shortest time possible. All plyometric exercises involve the stretch shortening cycle (SSC), which is a sequence of three phases (eccentric, amortization, and concentric). The first phase, eccentric, involves a quick stretch of the involved muscle. During this rapid stretch, energy is stored in elastic components of the musculotendinous structure and a stretch reflex is stimulated.

The next phase—ideally the shortest of the three phases—is the amortization phase. This phase is really a short pause to allow the reflexive nerve signals to communicate in the spinal cord before sending signals to the agonist muscle group. Lastly, the concentric phase is the payoff of the previous two phases. The energy stored in the elastic components is released and the nerve signal from the spinal reflex reaches the muscle. The result of these two components—release of stored elastic energy and spinal reflex—is an increase of force to a greater level than achieved by simple contraction alone. All three phases must occur for an exercise to be considered plyometric. The box jump is a common plyometric exercise because it involves all three SSC phases, whereas landing from a jump is not plyometric because the eccentric phase is essentially the only phase of the SSC occurring. Plyometric training as an injury prevention strategy is supported by several research studies and is included in most injury prevention programs, especially those designed to prevent ACL and ankle injuries.

Special Training

There are a variety of exercises that don't fall easily into strength or plyometric exercises, we have termed these special exercises. These exercises are more specific to an athlete's sport or position needs. These special exercises can be subdivided into three types of training: speed and agility, flexibility, and aerobic endurance.

Speed and Agility Training

Speed training involves the use of exercises to improve an athlete's movement velocity, whereas agility training uses exercises to improve an athlete's ability to change direction (typically in response to an external stimulus, like a defender). Both modes involve the use of rapid acceleration and the development of maximal force in the shortest time possible (i.e., RFD). Speed and agility training have direct application to injury prevention for many sports and body regions; speed training, as an example, should be a primary component of hamstring injury prevention programs and agility exercises are appropriate for all lower extremity injury prevention programs.

Flexibility Training

Flexibility is commonly defined as the range of motion of a joint. However, we do not believe range of motion alone adequately describes flexibility during sporting movements and therefore also include an assessment of muscle, tendon, and other tissue extensibility (i.e., the ability to be stretched). Consider the front split: Most people have the required range of joint motion in the hips to perform the front split, but still cannot perform the movement. The reason is not lack of range of motion; it is tissue extensibility, specifically of the hamstrings of the front leg and hip flexors of the trailing leg. Flexibility training, then, is the use of exercise to maximize both range of motion and tissue (primarily muscle) extensibility.

The two most common types of stretching are static and dynamic which both improve flexibility. Static stretching is passive in nature and involves holding a stretched position for a prolonged time. Dynamic stretching involves active movement while stretching. Both are commonly used during pregame warm-ups and postgame cool-downs. However, both are also somewhat controversial. Static stretching has been shown to significantly decrease power production for the short time after it has been performed (Opplert and Babault 2018; Sa et al. 2015; Yamaguchi et al. 2006). Further, there is little research to support the use of static or dynamic stretching to prevent injuries (Gremion 2005; Witvrouw et al. 2004).

Aerobic Endurance Training

Aerobic endurance training (also referred to as *cardiovascular* or *cardiorespiratory* training) is designed to improve the function of the cardiovascular and respiratory systems. There are several measurements used to assess this improvement (e.g., cardiac output, blood pressure, and minute ventilation), but the most commonly used measurement is maximal oxygen uptake ($\dot{V}O_2max$), or the maximal amount of oxygen that can be used by the cells in the body during exercise. Many training approaches can be used to improve $\dot{V}O_2max$, including the use of long slow distance, tempo, and interval training with different modes, like running, cycling, and swimming. Because fatigue has been described as a factor in athletic injuries, some suggest that athletes address this by training while in a fatigued state, but a better strategy may be to improve overall aerobic endurance in order to reduce the likelihood and intensity of fatigue.

ACTIVITY EXPOSURE

Participating in a physical activity over a prolonged period (i.e., several weeks or months) has the potential to reduce an athlete's risk of injury. This prolonged exposure to the physical stress of both training and practicing a sport is an important part of injury prevention training. Consider every college or professional sport; each of those athletes trains during the offseason (training exposure) and then participates in a preseason camp (practice exposure). This is an important combination of activities for those athletes as they prepare for games and competition.

One recent attempt to explain the benefits of this exposure has been the acute–chronic workload ratio (ACWR) (Gabbett et al. 2019; Johansson et al. 2022). The ACWR considers what an athlete has done in recent training, such as the past week (acute workload), in relation to what has been done over a longer period, such as the past month (chronic workload). It posits that, if the acute workload increases too much in relation to what has been done over the longer period of time, injury risk increases. Although several articles have been written about this topic, research is mixed as to the benefits of its use and fail to show that there is a specific ratio that should be followed for all athletes. However, we do generally believe that the greater exposure an athlete has to workloads over a longer period of time, the less likely she is to develop an injury.

Designing injury prevention programs requires knowledge of exercise principles to result in the best outcomes for the participating athletes. Exercises should have some similarity to the movements of the given sport or activity and the muscles should perform similar functions. A variety of exercise types must be included and they must be taught in ways that maximize movement success. Combining all of these is the fun part of designing injury prevention programs! In the following chapters, specific injury prevention exercises will be presented and both the anatomy of the specific muscles involved and the types of muscle contractions will be noted. Most importantly, each exercise will highlight a specific injury it can help prevent.

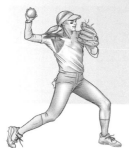

3

HEAD, NECK, AND SHOULDER

Injuries to the head, neck, and shoulders occur quite frequently in sport. Though closely related and interdependent, we have divided the discussion of these injuries into two general regions for ease of understanding: the head and neck (collectively) and the shoulder. Each of these regions will be discussed, and common injuries to each will be covered.

HEAD AND NECK

Several injuries can involve the head and neck, but we concentrate on two of the more common injuries: concussion and cervical (neck) muscle strain. Although these are different injuries, we have grouped them together because both respond well to exercises that focus on strengthening the muscles identified here. By strengthening these muscles, the neck becomes more stable and resistant to loads, and the risks of concussion and cervical muscle strain are decreased.

Concussion

Concussions are mild traumatic brain injuries that typically occur following a head impact; this impact results in the brain moving within—and hitting the sides of—the skull. Although there is no diagnostic test for a concussion, athletes with concussions may report various symptoms, including

- headache,
- impaired mental processes,
- increased irritability,
- forgetfulness,
- difficulty concentrating,
- loss of consciousness,
- nausea, and
- sleep disturbances.

Cervical Muscle Strain

Cervical muscle strains involve small tears in the muscles of the neck, which often occur when moving the neck through extreme ranges of motion or with excessive stress (either through overuse or a single event of overload). Athletes with cervical muscle strain commonly report symptoms such as general neck pain or stiffness, pain in the shoulders or upper back, muscle spasms, or headache, often starting at the base of the neck. In rare cases, athletes report numbness and tingling sensations in their upper extremities.

SHOULDER

The shoulder is the joint between the trunk and arm. The movements of the shoulder are accomplished by combinations of primarily posterior and anterior muscles that run between the trunk and the bones of the pectoral girdle and arm. One of the most mobile joints in the body, the shoulder allows us to carry objects, reach overhead, throw a ball, swim, and reach behind our backs. Accomplishing these tasks requires proper strength of several muscles to improve the stability of the shoulder joint. The shoulder is actually a combination of four primary joints: the glenohumeral joint, sternoclavicular joint, acromioclavicular joint, and scapulothoracic joint.

• *Glenohumeral joint.* This is the joint most people think of as "the shoulder." The glenohumeral joint is the articulation between the glenoid fossa of the scapula and the head of the humerus. This is most easily seen as the interaction of a ball in a socket (a concave area in which another object moves). Anatomically, the ball is the head of the humerus and the socket is the glenoid fossa (see figure 3.1). But, to function properly, the following three joints must also do their part.

• *Sternoclavicular joint.* The sternoclavicular joint allows small movement and is the articulation between the medial aspect of the clavicle and the superior portion of the sternum.

• *Acromioclavicular joint.* The acromioclavicular joint (sometimes referred to as the *AC joint*) also allows small movement and is the articulation between the lateral aspect of the clavicle and a portion of the scapula called the *acromion*.

• *Scapulothoracic joint.* The scapulothoracic joint is not a true articulation; rather, it is a functional joint between the anterior surface of the scapula and the posterior chest wall.

The large number of joints in the shoulder means a great amount of movement coordination is necessary, increasing the likelihood of injury. Further, because of the different types of joints involved, a variety of injuries can occur.

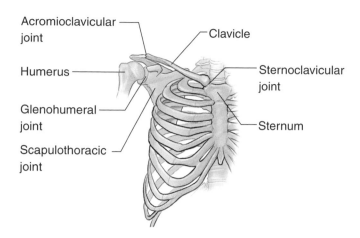

FIGURE 3.1   Joints of the shoulder: glenohumeral joint, sternoclavicular joint, acromioclavicular joint, and scapulothoracic joint.

Shoulder Impingement

Shoulder impingement is thought to occur when elevation of the arm (humerus) causes the head of the humerus to migrate superiorly (upward), thereby decreasing the space between the acromion and the humeral head. However, there has been recent debate regarding the use of this description as a cause of pain. Some have questioned whether the "pinching" during movement occurs and, if it does, if that indeed is the source of the pain. It is likely that other causes exist and that other structures are involved. Competing explanations for subacromial pain include tendinopathies of the rotator cuff muscles or simply increased sensitivity.

Rotator Cuff Strain

The rotator cuff is a group of four muscles and tendons—supraspinatus, infraspinatus, teres minor, and subscapularis—that help keep the head of the humerus centered in the glenoid fossa (see figure 3.2). Tendons of the rotator cuff surround the humeral head anteriorly, superiorly, and posteriorly, essentially becoming "dynamic ligaments" to improve glenohumeral stability. The socket of the joint (glenoid fossa) is very small and shallow compared to the size of the ball (humeral head). The rotator cuff muscles act to pull the head of the humerus medially into the glenoid fossa, providing most of the force resisting disarticulation (separation) of the joint. The active contraction of these muscles produces movement at the joint. Depending on the orientation of the glenohumeral joint, all rotator cuff muscles can rotate the humerus.

A strain, by definition, is the tearing of muscle fibers. Sometimes this tearing is mild (grade I), sometimes it involves a complete rupture (grade III),

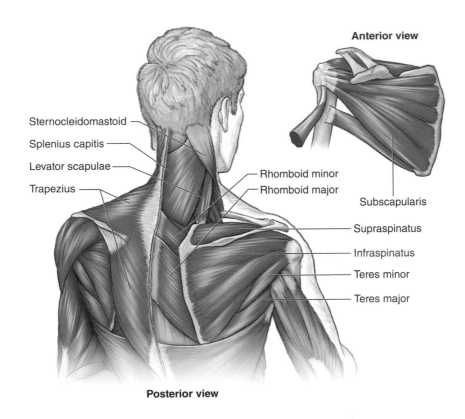

Anterior view

Sternocleidomastoid

Splenius capitis

Levator scapulae

Trapezius

Rhomboid minor

Rhomboid major

Subscapularis

Supraspinatus

Infraspinatus

Teres minor

Teres major

Posterior view

FIGURE 3.2   The muscles of the rotator cuff and the scapular stabilizing musculature.

and sometimes it is in between those two (grade II). Any of the rotator cuff muscles can become strained, often through overuse. The most frequently strained rotator cuff tendon is the supraspinatus.

Anterior Shoulder Instability

Of the four joints that make up the shoulder joint (see figure 3.1), the one that is most commonly susceptible to instability is the glenohumeral joint. Instability of this joint can result in a shoulder dislocation or subluxation, meaning the humeral head is no longer resting in the glenoid fossa. This dislocation typically occurs in an anterior direction, but it can occur in any direction.

CERVICAL ISOMETRIC—FLEXION

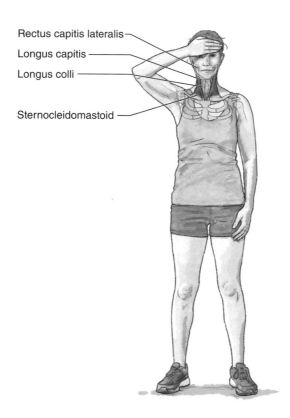

Rectus capitis lateralis
Longus capitis
Longus colli

Sternocleidomastoid

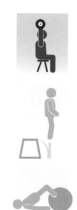

Execution

1. To improve alignment, start by looking straight ahead with your head level. Place one hand on your forehead to act as resistance.

2. Keeping your hand on your forehead, attempt to tilt your chin toward your chest. The hand on your forehead will prevent this motion, making the cervical muscles act isometrically. You may push as hard as is comfortable.

3. Maintain tension for 5 seconds, then relax.

Muscles Involved

Primary: Sternocleidomastoid

Secondary: Longus capitis, longus colli, rectus capitis anterior, rectus capitis lateralis

(continued)

CERVICAL ISOMETRIC—FLEXION   *(continued)*

PREVENTIVE FOCUS

When dysfunction of the cervical flexor muscles occurs, neck pain can occur and function (or even cognition) can be decreased. Use of the cervical muscles influences overall function by improving stability and control of the neck. Endurance of these muscles is important during both daily and sporting tasks.

Because it is quite difficult to isolate single muscles from the combined structures that support both the head and the neck, it is common for exercises that improve the function of this area to involve several muscles. The exercises described here all help to strengthen the identified muscles, thereby improving cervical stability and decreasing the risk of concussions and cervical muscle strains.

The cervical isometric exercises prevent injuries in a number of sports.

• Cycling on the road places a strain on all cervical muscles, but because the cyclist spends the majority of his time with the neck in an extended position, muscular endurance of the cervical extenders is important. However, if that is the only focus, the other muscles of the neck—such as sternocleidomastoid—become relatively underdeveloped, which can lead to pain and dysfunction.

• Wrestling requires the athlete to have his neck moved to extremes of flexion, extension, side bending, and rotation; therefore, it is essential that the muscles on all sides of the neck are strong enough to tolerate being placed in those severe positions without injuring the cervical spine.

• Football players of all positions rely on the strength of the cervical muscles to withstand the impact and heavy stresses involved with their sport, particularly tackling. During a tackle, the possibility of the head and neck experiencing sudden movement in an unexpected direction is very high. Rule changes and a greater focus on protecting the head and neck have helped, but because each play has a great degree of unpredictability, those rules cannot completely protect the players. Strengthening the muscles that surround the cervical spine is important for these athletes to reduce the risk of injury.

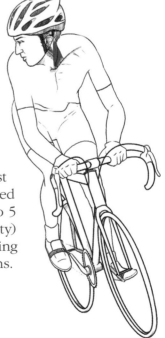

• Though not as popular a sport as others, auto racing requires special mention. Drivers must have sufficient cervical strength to tolerate prolonged high stresses. Drivers experience an average 4 to 5 g's (meaning four to five times the pull of gravity) during a race, which can peak to over 8 g's during tight turns, heavy braking, and rapid accelerations.

VARIATIONS

Cervical Isometric—Extension

To improve alignment, start by looking straight ahead with your head level. Place one hand on the back of your head to act as resistance.

Keeping your hand on the back of your head, attempt to look up at the ceiling. The hand on the back of your head will prevent this motion, making the cervical muscles act isometrically. You may push as hard as is comfortable.

Maintain tension for 5 seconds, then relax. The muscles involved with this variation differ from those used for flexion; specifically, splenius capitis and semispinalis capitis are the primary muscles, with trapezius assisting.

Cervical Isometric—Side Bending

To improve alignment, start by looking straight ahead with your head level. Place your hand on the side of your head just in front of your ear to act as resistance.

Keeping your hand on the side of your head, attempt to tilt your head toward that shoulder. The hand on the side of your head will prevent this motion, making the cervical muscles act isometrically. You may push as hard as is comfortable.

Maintain tension for 5 seconds, then relax. The muscles involved in this variation are similar to those used for flexion; specifically, sternocleidomastoid is the primary muscle, with splenius capitis, splenius cervicis, and scalenes (anterior, middle, posterior) assisting.

HEAD AND NECK

PUSH-UP WITH PLUS

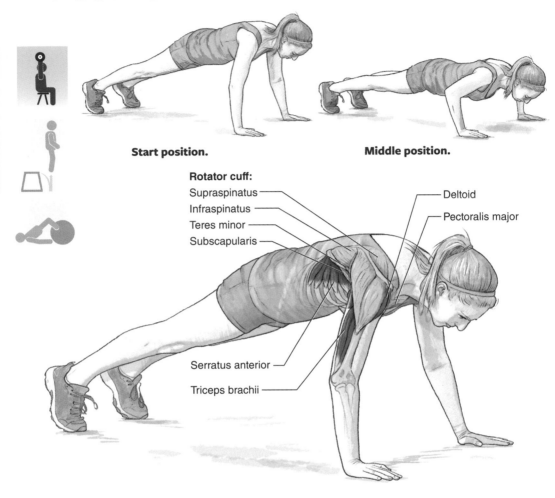

Start position.

Middle position.

Rotator cuff:
Supraspinatus
Infraspinatus
Teres minor
Subscapularis

Deltoid

Pectoralis major

Serratus anterior

Triceps brachii

Execution

1. Assume the standard push-up position with hands on the floor shoulder-width apart and the elbows, knees, and body straight.

2. Lower your body by allowing your elbows to flex and shoulders to horizontally abduct. Keep the body and knees straight during this movement. Continue lowering as deeply as possible without causing shoulder pain.

3. Raise your body by extending your elbows and horizontally adducting your shoulders. Keep the body and knees straight during this movement. Continue raising until your elbows are almost straight.

4. The "plus" portion of the exercise is accomplished by exaggerating the top position of the push-up. Keep your elbows straight but try to push your body up farther by separating your shoulder blades without rounding your back.

Muscles Involved

Primary: Pectoralis major, deltoid (primarily anterior), triceps brachii, serratus anterior

Secondary: Rotator cuff (supraspinatus, infraspinatus, teres minor, sub-scapularis)

PREVENTIVE FOCUS

The push-up is an excellent way to coordinate all four shoulder joints into one exercise. There are many variations, but the one best able to reduce injury risk is the push-up with plus. This variation is the standard push-up performed with an exaggerated motion at the top of the movement. The extra motion—scapular protraction—allows the serratus anterior to contribute to the exercise in a more pronounced fashion, thereby decreasing the risk of shoulder impingement.

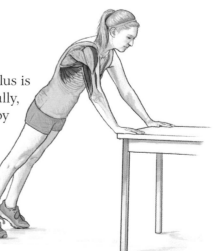

Strong shoulders are important for many sports, but especially so for throwing athletes. Although the motion of a push-up is similar to that of throwing, the most important benefit of the push-up with plus is the stability required to perform this motion, which requires the humeral head to move within the glenoid fossa. Further, push-ups generally require stability of the scapulae to correctly perform but adding the "plus" protraction action amplifies this requirement. If the throwing athlete does not have a strong base (scapulae), the likelihood for injury elsewhere (e.g., glenohumeral joint) increases. This does not mean the scapulae shouldn't move; it means the scapulae must move in a controlled manner that allows the other joints to also function properly.

VARIATION

Elevated Push-Up With Plus

The most common way to vary the push-up with plus is by changing the placement of the hands. Specifically, the intensity of the exercise can be decreased by moving the hands off the floor onto an elevated surface, such as a tabletop or countertop. The exercise is performed the same way and the same muscles are involved, but the intensity decreases because the effects of gravity are diminished.

DUMBBELL SHOULDER PRESS

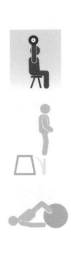

SHOULDER

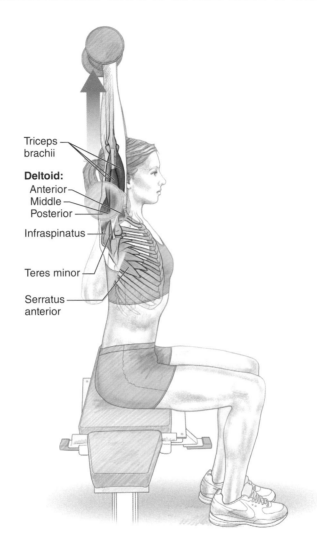

Triceps brachii

Deltoid:
Anterior
Middle
Posterior

Infraspinatus

Teres minor

Serratus anterior

Execution

1. Sit on a bench and place both feet on the floor.
2. Grasp the dumbbells with a closed, pronated grip.
3. Press the dumbbells over your head until your elbows are fully extended.
4. Keeping your forearms parallel, slowly flex your elbows to lower the dumbbells.
5. Lower the dumbbells until they touch your clavicles and front of the shoulders.
6. Do not arch the back.

Muscles Involved

Primary: Deltoid (anterior, middle, posterior), triceps brachii

Secondary: Rotator cuff (supraspinatus, infraspinatus, teres minor, sub-scapularis), trapezius, levator scapula, rhomboids, serratus anterior

PREVENTIVE FOCUS

Like the push-up with plus, the dumbbell shoulder press is a multijoint exercise that involves all four joints of the shoulder. This exercise is well suited to improve rotator cuff function and reduce injury risk. Note, however, that this is an advanced exercise—as discussed in previous chapters, you should begin with light resistance and increase as you are able.

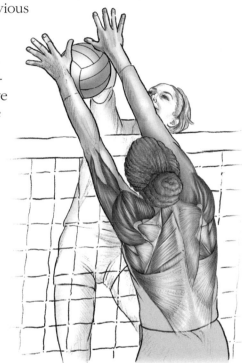

The dumbbell shoulder press is an important exercise for all overhead athletes. Overhead athletes require repeated movement above the level of their shoulders. Examples include swimmers, tennis players, baseball pitchers, and softball players. Volleyball players in particular—especially hitters and blockers—require strength in a fully flexed shoulder position (i.e., overhead). Because the highest position in the dumbbell shoulder press is similar to the position of a blocker at the net and to the hitting position when the player makes contact with the ball, this exercise specifically strengthens the upper extremity to tolerate those stresses and therefore reduce the player's risk of shoulder injury.

VARIATION

Barbell Shoulder Press

The most common way to vary the shoulder press is by using a barbell instead of dumbbells. Press the barbell overhead until your elbows are fully extended. Keeping your forearms parallel, slowly flex your elbows to lower the barbell. One other common variation involves moving the dumbbells or barbell behind the head. However, this variation should only be performed by experienced lifters because it can cause irritation to the front (anterior) of the shoulder, especially for those without significant weight training experience.

DUMBBELL ROW

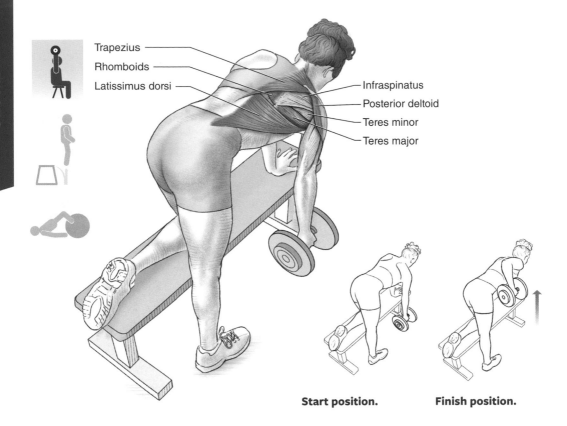

Trapezius

Rhomboids

Latissimus dorsi

Infraspinatus

Posterior deltoid

Teres minor

Teres major

Start position.   **Finish position.**

Execution

1. Position your right foot on the floor with the knee slightly flexed and place your left knee on a bench.
2. Rest your left hand on the bench.
3. Create a flat-back position with your torso parallel to the floor.
4. Grasp the dumbbell in your right hand with a closed, neutral grip.
5. Pull the dumbbell toward your torso, keeping your elbow close to the body.
6. Maintain your torso position with the right knee slightly flexed.
7. Touch the dumbbell to your lower chest or upper abdomen.
8. Lower the dumbbell back to the starting position.

Muscles Involved

Primary: Latissimus dorsi, teres major, trapezius, rhomboids, posterior deltoid

Secondary: Rotator cuff (supraspinatus, infraspinatus, teres minor, sub-scapularis), brachialis, biceps brachii

PREVENTIVE FOCUS

An exercise that involves all four joints of the shoulder, the dumbbell row is able to help reduce the risk of several injuries, including rotator cuff strain, shoulder instability, and shoulder impingement.

The most obvious application for the dumbbell row is crew; the upper extremity motion of rowing the shell is indeed similar to that of the dumbbell row. However, the power for the stroke in rowing is primarily generated from the lower extremities. An athlete who will benefit more from this exercise is a swimmer. The repeated motion of the shoulders for all strokes requires the muscles that surround the joints (i.e., glenohumeral and scapulothoracic) to be powerful but to also possess muscular endurance. The dumbbell row helps to improve both of these qualities and ultimately reduces injury risk as a result.

VARIATION

Barbell Bent-Over Row

The row can also be performed with a barbell in a bent-over position. This exercise involves the same muscles as the dumbbell row but also requires the stabilizers of the low back to become involved. For the barbell bent-over row, bend your torso forward in a flat-back position and hold the barbell with elbows fully extended. Pull the barbell toward your abdomen, then lower until the elbows are again fully extended.

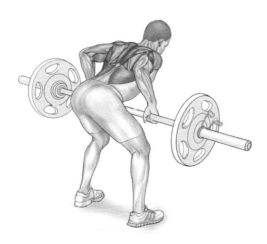

FARMER'S CARRY

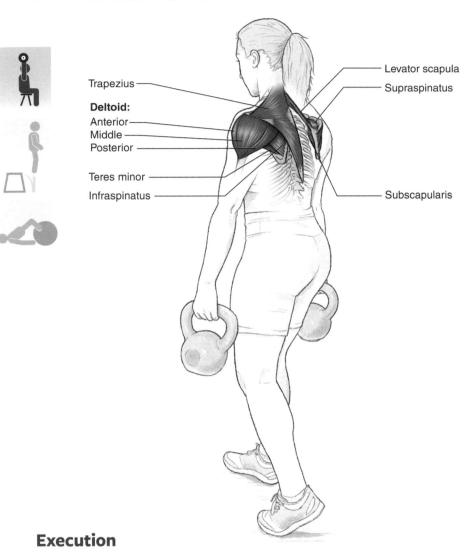

Trapezius

Deltoid:
Anterior
Middle
Posterior

Teres minor

Infraspinatus

Levator scapula

Supraspinatus

Subscapularis

Execution

1. From a standing position, grasp a kettlebell in each hand with a closed, pronated grip.
2. Hold the kettlebells at your sides with elbows extended.
3. Maintaining this position, walk for a specified distance.

Muscles Involved

Primary and secondary: Rotator cuff (supraspinatus, infraspinatus, teres minor, subscapularis), trapezius, levator scapulae, deltoid (anterior, middle, posterior)

Note: Although the muscles of the lower extremities and forearm play a primary role in this exercise, we will focus on the shoulder muscles involved here, which act isometrically to maintain joint alignment.

PREVENTIVE FOCUS

The farmer's carry is used in strongman competitions, but it is a very good exercise to develop the stabilizers of the glenohumeral joint (and grip and even low back) and improve strength endurance of the involved muscles. By involving all rotator cuff muscles, it is a good choice for reducing the risk of both rotator cuff strain and shoulder instability episodes.

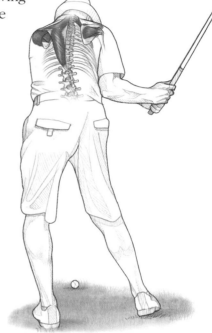

The farmer's carry has multiple purposes for both performance training and injury prevention. It is included in the shoulder section because it requires all of the rotator cuff muscles to function. This is important during activities that require shoulder stability—for example, golf. When swinging, the muscles for the lead shoulder undergo a strong eccentric contraction followed almost immediately by a forceful concentric contraction. Using an exercise that strengthens the rotator cuff muscles for this type of movement is important.

VARIATION

Unstable Farmer's Carry

Common variations of the farmer's carry include using unstable or variable resistances, such as walking uphill or carrying fluid-filled buckets.

PRONE HORIZONTAL ABDUCTION

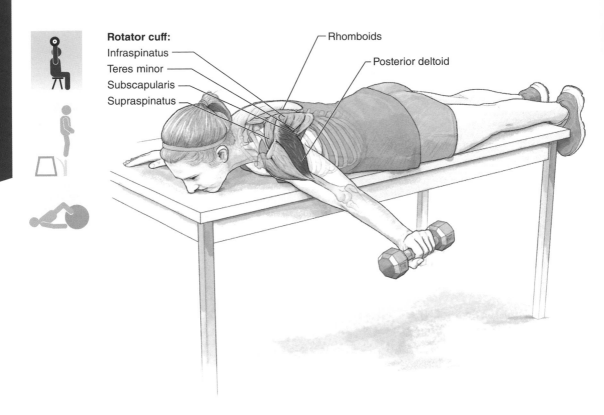

Rotator cuff:
Infraspinatus
Teres minor
Subscapularis
Supraspinatus

Rhomboids

Posterior deltoid

Execution

1. Lie prone on a bed or table with one arm hanging straight down off the side, perpendicular to the floor.
2. Grasp a dumbbell in that hand, with the thumb facing forward.
3. Keeping your elbow extended, raise the hanging arm straight out to the side until it is parallel to the floor. (At this position, your arm is at 90 degrees to your torso and your palm is facing the floor.)
4. Slowly lower your arm to the hanging position.

Muscles Involved

Primary: Deltoid (posterior)

Secondary: Rotator cuff (supraspinatus, infraspinatus, teres minor, subscapularis), rhomboids

PREVENTIVE FOCUS

Prone horizontal abduction is a challenging single-joint exercise that does not require heavy weight to be effective. Prone horizontal abduction helps to reduce shoulder impingement and rotator cuff strain.

This and the following three exercises—termed *shoulder isolation exercises*—target the rotator cuff in a variety of ways. Some isolate specific muscles (e.g., external rotation at 90 degrees), whereas some require the rotator cuff to work with other motions (e.g., D2 flexion with band). But all of these exercises rely on the rotator cuff to help maintain the position of the humeral head in the glenoid fossa at extremes of available joint motion with ballistic activities, when decelerating the arm, when hanging, and with impact. Examples include throwing, tennis, gymnastics, and obstacle course racing.

VARIATION

Prone Horizontal Abduction at 100 Degrees

By changing the angle and rotation of the arm, the exercise can change its focus. The most common variation is performing the exercise in an externally rotated position, at an angle just greater than the typical execution. Specifically, your palm will face forward and your arm will be at 100 degrees to your torso at the top position. This then tends to involve the supraspinatus to a greater degree.

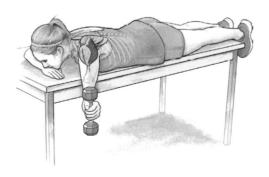

SCAPTION

SHOULDER

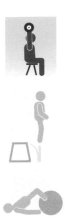

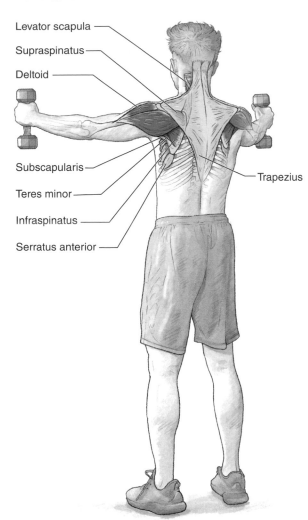

Levator scapula

Supraspinatus

Deltoid

Subscapularis

Teres minor

Infraspinatus

Serratus anterior

Trapezius

Execution

1. Stand with your feet shoulder- or hip-width apart and with your knees slightly flexed. Grasp a dumbbell in each hand with a closed, neutral grip.

2. Externally rotate your shoulders and then raise the dumbbells up and out to the sides at a 30-degree angle in front of the body. Your elbows and upper arms should rise together and ahead of the forearms and hands.

3. Continue raising the dumbbells until your arms are parallel to the floor or at shoulder level. Your thumb should be pointing up at the top position.

4. Slowly lower the dumbbells to the starting position.

Muscles Involved

Primary: Rotator cuff (infraspinatus, supraspinatus, subscapularis, teres minor), deltoid (anterior, middle, posterior)

Secondary: Trapezius, levator scapulae, serratus anterior

PREVENTIVE FOCUS

Also called the "full can," scaption involves abduction of the arm but at an angle in front of the body's plane—specifically, the scapular plane, which is 30 degrees anterior to the body's plane. Scaption helps to reduce shoulder impingement and rotator cuff strain. As with the previous exercise, this exercise is beneficial for athletes in several sports, including gymnasts.

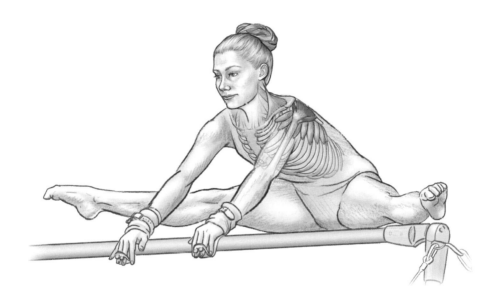

EXTERNAL ROTATION AT 90 DEGREES

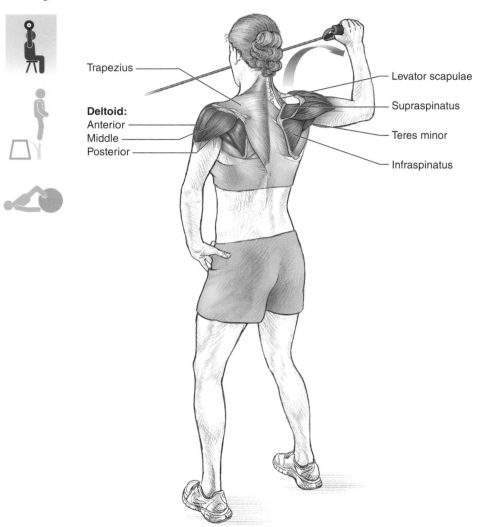

Trapezius

Deltoid:
Anterior
Middle
Posterior

Levator scapulae

Supraspinatus

Teres minor

Infraspinatus

Execution

Note: You will need an elastic cord or resistance band to perform this exercise.

1. Stand with your feet shoulder-width apart. With the other end fixed in front of you, grip the resistance band with your shoulder abducted to 90 degrees, elbow flexed at 90 degrees, and forearm parallel to the floor.

2. While maintaining the abducted shoulder position, externally rotate your shoulder (the elbow remains bent at 90 degrees).

3. Return the resistance band to the starting position (forearm parallel to the floor).

Muscles Involved

Primary: Supraspinatus, infraspinatus, teres minor, deltoid (anterior, middle, posterior)

Secondary: Trapezius, levator scapulae, subscapularis

PREVENTIVE FOCUS

Because the primary stabilizers of the shoulder joint are also involved in rotation at the glenohumeral joint, exercises that use this type of motion are important. External rotation at 90 degrees is a particularly effective exercise to help increase shoulder stability while reducing the risk of shoulder impingement and rotator cuff strain. As with the previous two exercises, this exercise is beneficial to athletes in several sports, including tennis players.

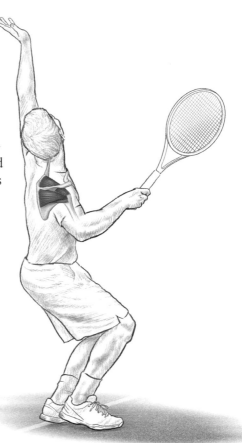

VARIATION

External Rotation at 90 Degrees— Fast

The most common way to vary external rotation at 90 degrees is by performing the exercise at an increased speed, which more closely mimics the required muscle action of throwing.

D2 FLEXION WITH BAND

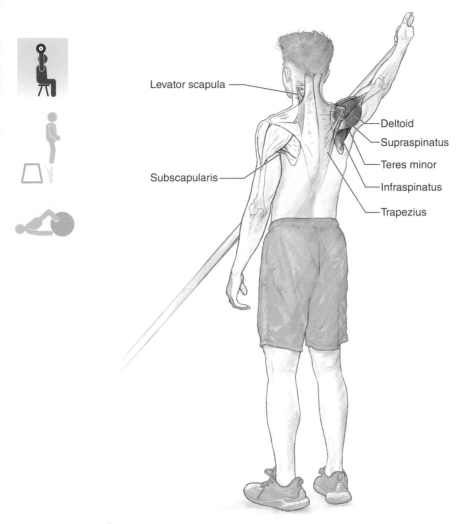

Levator scapula

Deltoid

Supraspinatus

Teres minor

Subscapularis

Infraspinatus

Trapezius

Execution

Note: You will need an elastic cord or resistance band to perform this exercise.

1. Stand with your feet shoulder-width apart. With one end of the elastic resistance band anchored in front of you and to the left, cross your right arm across your body and hold the other end of the band in your right hand near your left hip.

2. Keeping your elbow slightly flexed, externally rotate your right arm to lift it up to an overhead position.

3. Return the resistance band to the starting position by allowing your arm to internally rotate. An easy way to think of how to rotate your arm is that your thumb should lead the way: When lifting up, the thumb turns up; when returning to the starting position, the thumb turns down.

Muscles Involved

Primary: Supraspinatus, infraspinatus, teres minor, deltoid (anterior, middle, posterior)

Secondary: Trapezius, levator scapulae, subscapularis

PREVENTIVE FOCUS

Because most sporting movements involving the shoulder occur in multiple planes, it is important to include an exercise that targets this type of motion. D2 flexion helps to increase shoulder stability through shoulder flexion, abduction, horizontal abduction, and external rotation, thereby reducing the risk of shoulder impingement and rotator cuff strain. As with the previous exercise, this exercise is beneficial to athletes in several sports, especially those involving throwing.

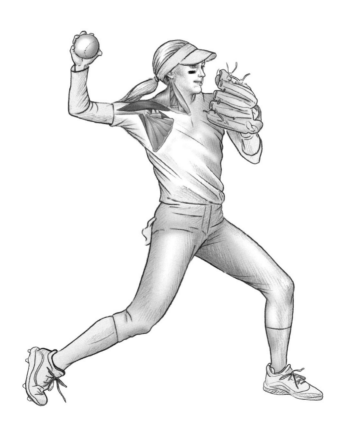

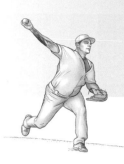

4

ELBOW, WRIST, AND HAND

In addition to the shoulder joint, injuries to the other structures of the upper extremity do occur in a variety of sports. Although several joints and structures exist, the upper extremity can be generally divided into three segments (the arm, the forearm, and the hand) connected at two joints (the elbow and the wrist). This chapter will specifically focus on the arm and elbow, the forearm and wrist, and the hand—the three areas most likely to be involved in sport-related injuries. The anatomy of each area will be presented, and discussion of common injuries will follow. However, this is a complex area of the body and although structures have been grouped in a specific manner, it should be noted that some muscles act on multiple joints.

ARM AND ELBOW

The anatomical *arm* is the area between the shoulder and elbow joint. The arm is composed of the humerus and can be divided into anterior and posterior compartments and the elbow joint includes three bones: the humerus, ulna, and radius. There are five muscles in the arm: three flexors in the anterior compartment and two extensors in the posterior compartment.

1. *Biceps brachii.* This is the most superficial muscle of the arm and, as its name indicates, it has two heads, the short head and the long head. Both heads have origins on the scapula (short head: coracoid process of scapula, long head: supraglenoid tubercle of the scapula) and join to insert on the radius at the radial tuberosity. Though typically considered a flexor of the elbow joint (a job it does assist with), the primary function of biceps brachii is to supinate the forearm, making supination a very strong motion compared to pronation. Interestingly, biceps brachii has no real attachment to the humerus (see figure 4.1).

2. *Brachialis.* Brachialis has an extensive origin from the anterior aspect of the distal half of the humerus and inserts on the ulna at the coronoid process and tuberosity. Its only action is flexion of the forearm (see figure 4.1).

3. *Coracobrachialis.* Coracobrachialis originates on the coracoid process of the scapula and inserts on the middle third of the medial surface of the humerus. It assists with flexion and adduction of the humerus and helps to stabilize the shoulder joint.

4. *Triceps brachii.* This is the primary muscle of the posterior arm and has three heads: long, lateral, and medial (see figure 4.2). The long head originates on the infraglenoid tubercle of the scapula, the lateral head originates on the posterior surface of humerus, and the medial head originates on the posterior surface of humerus; all three join to insert on the proximal end of olecranon process of the ulna. Triceps brachii extends the forearm but, through the long head's attachment to the scapulae, also steadies the head of the humerus when the shoulder is in abduction.

5. *Anconeus.* This small muscle originates on the lateral epicondyle of humerus and inserts on the lateral surface of ulna's olecranon process. It assists the triceps in extending the forearm and stabilizes the elbow joint. While it is listed separately, the anconeus should functionally be considered a part of triceps brachii and not a separate functional muscle.

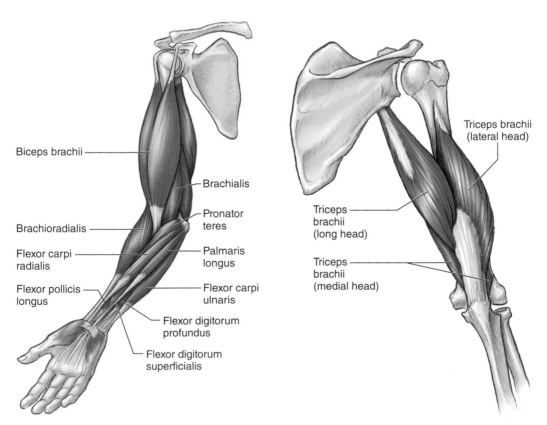

FIGURE 4.1 Upper extremity anatomy.

FIGURE 4.2 Triceps brachii muscle.

Though correctly understood as a hinge joint, the elbow is a complex joint between the distal end of the humerus and the proximal ends of the ulna and radius. The elbow primarily allows for the flexion and extension of the forearm, but it does move medially and laterally to much lesser degrees. The injuries that occur at the elbow can happen in a number of ways and can involve multiple structures. Ligaments, bones, muscles, and tendons are all structures that are commonly injured at the elbow joint.

A special note about the wrist extensors and flexors: Because these muscles primarily function at the wrist joint, they are covered in a subsequent section. However, many of these muscles originate on the humerus and have a role at the elbow. Further, when injured, the pain and dysfunction experienced may be near the elbow. Therefore, it is important to acknowledge these muscles in this section, though they are more traditionally viewed as muscles that provide movement at the wrist joint.

Ulnar Collateral Sprain

One of the most researched injuries to the elbow joint is a sprain of the ulnar collateral ligament (UCL). The UCL resists valgus elbow forces, which push the forearm laterally (out) relative to the arm. Although these forces don't occur during most daily activities, they are common when throwing, as in baseball and softball. This throwing motion results in increased tension in the medial structures of the elbow, specifically the UCL. When the tension is combined with the rapid acceleration of the upper extremity during a throw, tearing of the UCL fibers can occur, which may result in a sprain. If the fibers are torn to a great enough degree to cause instability, surgery can be indicated; the common surgical technique is UCL reconstruction, commonly referred to as *Tommy John surgery.*

Little League Elbow

This injury is common in younger, skeletally immature throwers who have open growth plates. In some ways, it is similar to the UCL sprain because the mechanism is essentially the same. Instead of the ligamentous fibers tearing, however, the open growth plate can become damaged or the UCL can pull away from its attachment to the humerus at the medial epicondyle.

Lateral Epicondylitis

Lateral epicondylitis occurs when forearm extensor tendons that attach to the humerus are overloaded and irritation with potential microtearing can occur. Though commonly referred to as *tennis elbow,* this injury can occur in a variety of sports, particularly those with repetitive gripping and with elbow and wrist motions. The forearm muscles and tendons become damaged from the overuse of repeated motions or activities.

Medial Epicondylitis

Medial epicondylitis—commonly referred to as *golfer's elbow*—is an injury of the wrist flexors near their attachment on the medial epicondyle of the humerus. This is an overload injury of the tendon following repetitive forced, passive wrist extension, and forearm supination, leading to degeneration. Activities that can result in this include those involving wrist flexion and forearm pronation.

Triceps and Biceps Tendinopathies

Irritation of the triceps tendon as it inserts into the olecranon process is termed *triceps tendinopathy*, or weightlifter's elbow. Irritation of this tendon is typically caused by repeated motion—specifically extension—at the elbow. Throwing, push-ups, bench press, and other activities that involve a lot of force development in the triceps are motions that can lead to injury of the triceps tendon.

Biceps tendinopathy commonly involves the tendon of the long head of the biceps brachii muscle, but can also involve its distal insertion on the radius. Long head tendinopathy is commonly considered a shoulder injury because this tendon attaches to the supraglenoid tubercle of the scapulae. This proximal biceps injury is common with the repetitive motions of overhead athletes, like swimming, volleyball, tennis, and throwing sports. Although repetitive motion can cause distal biceps tendinopathy, it is more likely caused by lifting a weight that is too heavy. Injury to the distal biceps brachii tendon is not common.

FOREARM AND WRIST

The forearm is the area between the elbow and wrist joints. The forearm comprises the radius and ulna and can be divided into anterior and posterior compartments, though these are more commonly referred to as *flexor* and *extensor* compartments, respectively (see figure 4.3). There are many muscles in the forearm; please refer to tables 4.1 and 4.2 for a complete list.

The wrist is a complex combination of several joints between the forearm and the hand. The bones of this joint are arranged in two rows, collectively known as the carpal bones. The proximal row comprises scaphoid, lunate, triquetrum, and pisiform; the distal row comprises trapezium, trapezoid, capitate, and hamate.

- *Radiocarpal joint.* This joint is the articulation between the distal end of the radius and the proximal row of the carpal bones.
- *Midcarpal joint.* This joint is the articulation between the proximal and distal rows of carpal bones.
- *Carpometacarpal joint.* This joint is the articulation between the proximal end of the metacarpal bones and the surfaces of the distal row of the carpal bones. The carpometacarpal joint of the thumb is the articulation between the trapezium to the first metacarpal bone; it is sometimes considered a different joint because its function differs from the other four carpometacarpal joints.

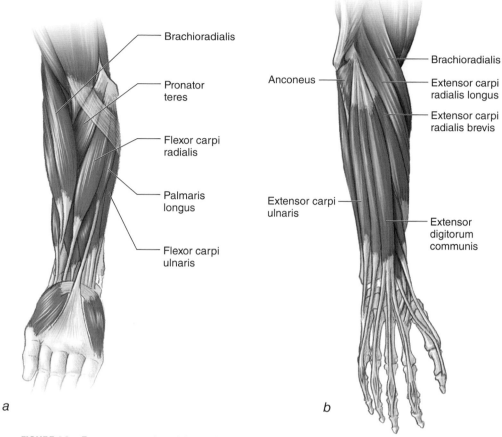

FIGURE 4.3 Forearm muscles: *(a)* anterior and *(b)* posterior.

TABLE 4.1 Flexor Muscles of the Forearm

MUSCLE	ORIGIN	INSERTION	ACTION
PRONATOR TERES	Common flexor tendon (medial epicondyle of humerus)	Middle of lateral surface of radius	Pronation and some flexion of forearm
FLEXOR CARPI RADIALIS	Common flexor tendon (medial epicondyle of humerus)	Base of second metacarpal bone	Flexion and abduction of wrist
PALMARIS LONGUS	Common flexor tendon (medial epicondyle of humerus)	Palmar aponeurosis	Flexion of wrist
FLEXOR CARPI ULNARIS	Common flexor tendon (medial epicondyle of humerus)	Pisiform bone (palmar surface); hook of hamate bone (palmar surface); fifth metacarpal bone	Flexion and abduction of wrist

(continued)

TABLE 4.1   Flexor Muscles of the Forearm *(continued)*

MUSCLE	ORIGIN	INSERTION	ACTION
FLEXOR DIGITORUM SUPERFICIALIS	Common flexor tendon (medial epicondyle of humerus); superior half of anterior radius	Medial four digits	Flexion of middle four phalanges of medial four digits
FLEXOR DIGITORUM PROFUNDUS	Proximal 3/4 of medial and anterior surfaces of ulna	Base of the distal phalanx of digits 2-5	Flexion of distal phalanges of medial four digits and assistance with wrist flexion
FLEXOR POLLICIS LONGUS	Anterior surface of radius	Base of distal phalanx of thumb	Flexion of thumb phalanges
PRONATOR QUADRATUS	Distal 1/4 of anterior surface of ulna	Distal 1/4 of anterior surface of radius	Pronation of forearm

TABLE 4.2   Extensor Muscles of the Forearm

MUSCLE	ORIGIN	INSERTION	ACTION
BRACHIORADIALIS	Upper 2/3 of supracondylar ridge of humerus	Styloid process of radius	Flexion of forearm when forearm is pronated
EXTENSOR CARPI RADIALIS LONGUS	Lateral supracondylar ridge (of humerus)	Base of second metacarpal bone	Extension of wrist and abduction of hand at the wrist
EXTENSOR CARPI RADIALIS BREVIS	Common extensor tendon (lateral epicondyle of humerus)	Base of third metacarpal bone	Extension of wrist and abduction of hand at the wrist
EXTENSOR DIGITORUM COMMUNIS	Common extensor tendon (lateral epicondyle of humerus)	Medial four digits	Extension of fingers and wrist
EXTENSOR DIGITI MINIMI	Common extensor tendon (lateral epicondyle of humerus)	Fifth digit	Independent extension of the fifth digit
EXTENSOR CARPI ULNARIS	Common extensor tendon (lateral epicondyle of humerus)	Base of fifth metacarpal	Adduction of wrist and assistance with wrist extension
SUPINATOR	Lateral epicondyle of humerus	Lateral, posterior, and anterior surfaces of upper 1/3 of radius	Supination of forearm and assistance of biceps brachii with forearm supination
ABDUCTOR POLLICIS LONGUS	Posterior surfaces of ulna and radius	Base of first metacarpal	Abduction of thumb and extension of thumb at carpometacarpal joint
EXTENSOR POLLICIS BREVIS	Posterior surfaces of radius	Base of proximal phalanx of thumb	Extension of proximal phalanx of thumb at carpometacarpal joint
EXTENSOR POLLICIS LONGUS	Posterior surface of middle 1/3 of ulna	Base of distal phalanx of thumb	Extension of distal phalanx of thumb at carpometacarpal and interphalangeal joints
EXTENSOR INDICIS	Posterior surface of ulna	Extensor expansion of second digit	Extension of second digit and assistance with hand extension

- *Distal radioulnar joint.* This is a pivot-type joint between the radius and the ulna just proximal to the wrist joint; motions here include pronation and supination of the forearm.

Fractures to the bones of the wrist are common but are difficult to prevent. Most injuries that occur at the wrist involve overuse or repetitive strains; these are the types of injuries that respond best to injury prevention.

Flexor Muscle Strain

Irritation of the wrist flexor and pronator muscles distal (beyond) to the medial epicondyle is termed *flexor muscle strain* (not to be confused with golfer's elbow, which occurs at the medial epicondyle). This injury involves the muscle belly and not the common flexor tendon's insertion into the medial epicondyle. Athletes who throw or use repeated wrist and forearm motion are at risk for this injury.

Wrist Ligament Sprain or Strain

Injury to any of the several ligaments stabilizing the wrist is termed a *sprain*. Wrist ligament sprains are typically due to repeated motions and overuse. Throwing or gripping may also cause wrist pain, which often increases after prolonged or repeated movements.

HAND

The hand is the area distal to the wrist joint and comprises 19 bones. There are several extrinsic and intrinsic muscles that help the hand function. The extrinsic muscles, listed in the forearm and wrist section, are those that originate in the forearm. These muscles assist with hand function, but also play important roles at the wrist. The intrinsic muscles consist of smaller muscles that originate and insert within the hand and are responsible for functions such as pinch and grip. Like the forearm, there are great number of intrinsic hand muscles (see figure 4.4 and table 4.3).

The hand has many similarities from finger to finger. There are five metacarpal bones that articulate with the wrist at the carpometacarpal joints. Each metacarpal bone connects to one finger—or phalanx—at the metacarpophalangeal (MCP) joint. Each finger has three individual phalanges separated by two interphalangeal joints—a proximal interphalangeal (PIP) joint and a distal interphalangeal (DIP) joint. The thumb has two phalanges and one interphalangeal (IP) joint.

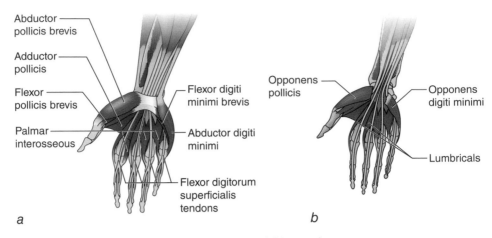

FIGURE 4.4   Intrinsic hand muscles: *(a)* anterior and *(b)* posterior.

TABLE 4.3   Intrinsic Muscles of the Hand

MUSCLE	ORIGIN	INSERTION	ACTION
ABDUCTOR POLLICIS BREVIS	Flexor retinaculum and tubercle of scaphoid	Lateral aspect of proximal phalanx of thumb	Abduction of thumb
FLEXOR POLLICIS BREVIS	Flexor retinaculum and tubercle of trapezium	Lateral aspect of proximal phalanx of thumb	Flexion of thumb
OPPONENS POLLICIS	Flexor retinaculum and tubercle of trapezium	Lateral aspect of thumb	Opposition of thumb
ABDUCTOR DIGITI MINIMI	Pisiform	Medial aspect of the proximal phalanx of fifth digit	Abduction of fifth digit
FLEXOR DIGITI MINIMI BREVIS	Flexor retinaculum and hook of the hamate	Medial aspect of the proximal phalanx of the fifth digit	Flexion of fifth digit
OPPONENS DIGITI MINIMI	Flexor retinaculum and hook of the hamate	Medial aspect of the fifth metacarpal	Opposition of fifth digit
DORAL INTEROSSEI MUSCLES	Metacarpals	Extensor hood and proximal phalanges of digits 2-4	Abduction of digits 2-4
PALMAR INTEROSSEI MUSCLES	Palmar aspect of metacarpals 2, 4, 5	Extensor hood and proximal phalanges of digits 2, 4, 5	Adduction of digits 2-4
LUMBRICALS	Tendons of flexor digitorum profundus	Extensor hood of digits 2-5	Flexion of MCP joints with extension of PIP and DIP joints

MCP = metacarpophalangeal
PIP = proximal interphalangeal
DIP = distal interphalangeal

Most hand injuries are related specifically to the bones and involve crushing injuries, fractures, or avulsions. Some of these fractures are

- boxer's fracture (fracture of the fifth metatarsal),
- Bennett's fracture (fracture at the base of the thumb),
- Rolando's fracture (fracture and dislocation of the thumb),
- jersey finger avulsion (rupture of a flexor tendon from its insertion on the distal phalanx), and
- mallet finger avulsion (rupture of an extensor tendon from its insertion on the distal phalanx).

Although protective equipment is helpful, it is very difficult to use exercise to reduce the risk of these injuries.

Other hand injuries also involve tendons or ligaments. Three of the most common are de Quervain's tenosynovitis, gamekeeper's thumb, and skier's thumb.

de Quervain's Tenosynovitis

de Quervain's tenosynovitis is an overuse injury to the abductor pollicis longus and extensor pollicis brevis tendons. Specific activities that can cause this include "wringing a washcloth, gripping a golf club, lifting a child, or hammering a nail" (Goel and Abzug, 2015).

Gamekeeper's Thumb and Skier's Thumb

Both of these terms refer to an avulsion or rupture of the ulnar collateral ligament (UCL) of the first metacarpophalangeal joint. The difference between the two involves the way the UCL was damaged; gamekeeper's thumb is an overuse injury to the UCL, whereas skier's thumb is an acute UCL injury due to hyperabduction of the thumb as it is caught by the ski pole strap.

OVERHEAD TRICEPS EXTENSION

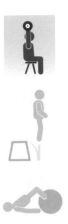

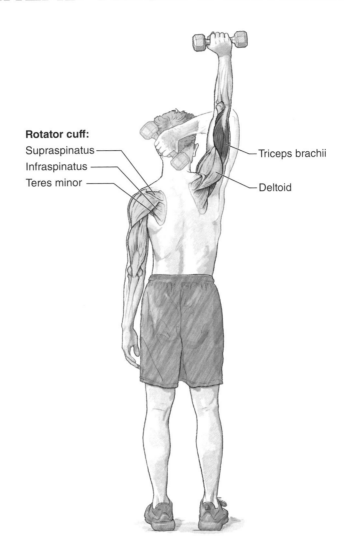

Rotator cuff:
Supraspinatus
Infraspinatus
Teres minor

Triceps brachii
Deltoid

Execution

1. Stand with your feet shoulder-width apart and your left arm to your side. Hold a dumbbell in your right hand with your right arm held behind the head and upper back and your elbow flexed.

2. Keeping your right wrist rigid, push the dumbbell upward until your elbow is fully extended.

3. Allow your right elbow to flex to slowly lower the dumbbell to the starting position.

4. At the completion of the set, repeat the movement with the other arm.

Muscles Involved

Primary: Triceps brachii

Secondary: Rotator cuff (supraspinatus, infraspinatus, teres minor, subscapularis), deltoid (anterior, middle, posterior)

PREVENTIVE FOCUS

Triceps injuries occur when a rapid force is applied through this muscle and its tendon, such as a throwing motion. Loading these structures helps to improve their strength, thereby reducing the likelihood of triceps muscle strain or tendinopathy.

Because of the rapid elbow extension, the overhead triceps extension is an important exercise for all throwing athletes, including shot putters, baseball pitchers, and softball players. One benefit of this exercise is improved performance, but another is reduced risk of injury. Because it involves the long head more than the standard triceps push-down exercise, the overhead triceps extension places a greater stretch on the triceps tendon, thereby increasing its ability to tolerate the throwing motion.

VARIATION

Triceps Kickback

Instead of standing with the dumbbell, the triceps kickback requires you to support your upper body on a bench. Bend forward slightly, keeping your upper body in alignment. Place one hand on the bench for support and hold the dumbbell in the other hand. Slowly extend your elbow back while keeping your upper arm in tight by your side.

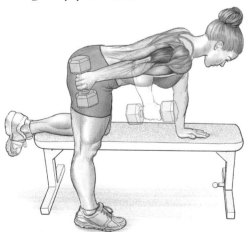

BARBELL BICEPS CURL

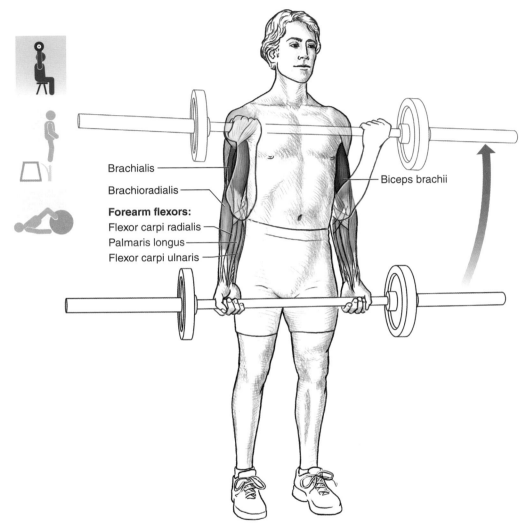

Brachialis

Brachioradialis

Biceps brachii

Forearm flexors:
Flexor carpi radialis
Palmaris longus
Flexor carpi ulnaris

Execution

1. Stand with your feet shoulder-width apart and grasp the bar with a closed, supinated grip, hands at or slightly wider than shoulder width.

2. Position the bar in front of your thighs with your elbows fully extended and upper arms against the sides of your torso, perpendicular to the floor.

3. Keeping your upper arms stationary, flex your elbows to move the bar toward your shoulders until the bar is within 4 to 6 inches (10-15 cm) of the shoulders.

4. Still keeping your upper arms stationary, allow your elbows to slowly extend back to the starting position.

Muscles Involved

Primary: Brachialis, biceps brachii

Secondary: Brachioradialis, forearm flexors (flexor carpi radialis, palmaris longus, flexor carpi ulnaris), supinator

PREVENTIVE FOCUS

Distal biceps brachii injuries typically occur when a large force is applied through the muscle and tendon, whereas proximal injuries typically occur during overhead activities. Loading these structures helps to improve their strength, thereby reducing the likelihood of biceps brachii muscle strain or tendinopathy. In addition, because this exercise loads the elbow joint, UCL injury risk is reduced.

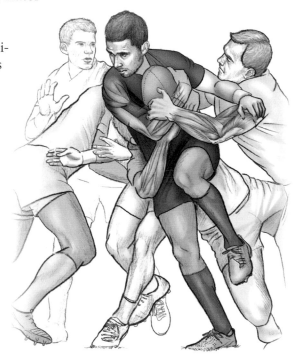

Two sports have unique requirements of the distal biceps brachii, and their athletes would benefit by incorporating the barbell biceps curl into their training:

• Rugby athletes often have the ball pulled out of their hands during play, which applies stress to the flexed elbow and increases the possibility of a distal biceps brachii injury. Strong elbow flexors (i.e., brachialis, biceps brachii) are needed to resist this motion. The barbell biceps curl can reduce the risk of this injury.

• Softball pitchers would also particularly benefit from the barbell biceps curl exercise. The underhand softball pitching motion requires forceful, repeated activity of brachialis and biceps brachii. To reduce a softball pitcher's risk of elbow or distal biceps tendon injury, incorporation of this exercise should be strongly considered.

VARIATION

Alternate Dumbbell Biceps Curl

Stand erect or sit on a weight bench as shown. Grasp a dumbbell in each hand with your thumbs toward the front. Keeping your arm next to your side, flex your right elbow and supinate (turn palm upward). Lower the dumbbell until your elbow is fully extended, allowing your forearm to pronate until your thumb is again toward the front. Repeat with other side.

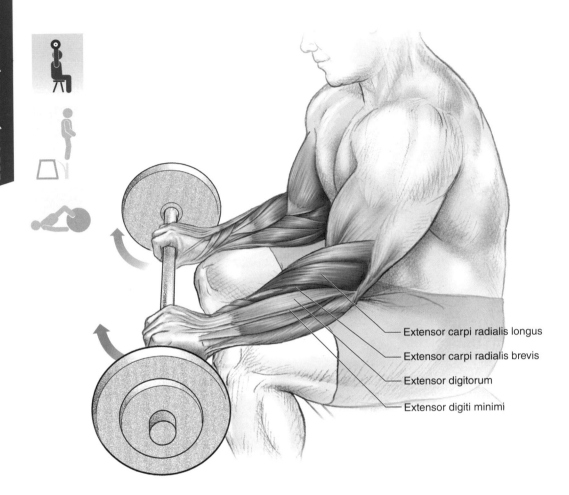

BARBELL WRIST EXTENSION

Extensor carpi radialis longus

Extensor carpi radialis brevis

Extensor digitorum

Extensor digiti minimi

Execution

1. Sit on a bench with your feet flat on the floor and grasp a bar with a closed, pronated grip, hands hip-width apart. Rest your elbows and forearms on top of your thighs with wrists and hands anterior to—or in front of—the knees.

2. Raise the bar up as far as possible by extending your wrists without moving your elbows or forearms.

3. Allow your wrists to slowly flex back to the starting position.

Muscles Involved

Primary: Extensor carpi radialis longus, extensor carpi radialis brevis

Secondary: Extensor digitorum, extensor digiti minimi, extensor indicis

PREVENTIVE FOCUS

Strengthening the wrist extensors—as with the barbell wrist extension—helps to stabilize the wrist joint and reduce the risk of injuries, including grip-related injuries that occur in sport and occupations that require repetitive grasping and gripping. Tennis is the most obvious example of a sport that would benefit from performing the barbell wrist extension. (As stated earlier, injury to the common extensor tendon is even termed *tennis elbow.*) Tennis involves two motions that require the wrist extensors to properly function: repeated gripping and resisted wrist extension. A strong correlation exists between grip strength and wrist extensor strength. Further, when hitting—especially with a backhand stroke—the wrist extensors resist flexion of the wrist to keep the wrist stable. By strengthening the wrist extensors, the risk of injury to the common extensor tendon at the lateral epicondyle lessens.

VARIATION

Standing Dumbbell Wrist Extension

Stand with your feet shoulder-width apart and grasp a dumbbell in each hand with a closed, pronated grip, elbows and forearms at your sides. Raise each dumbbell up as far as possible by extending your wrists without moving the elbows or forearms. Allow your wrists to slowly flex back to the starting position.

BARBELL WRIST FLEXION

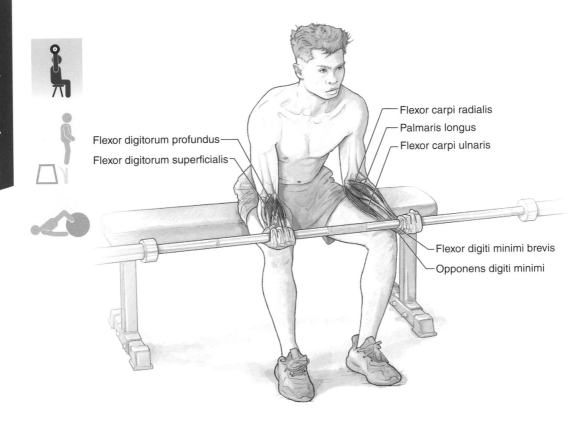

Flexor digitorum profundus
Flexor digitorum superficialis
Flexor carpi radialis
Palmaris longus
Flexor carpi ulnaris
Flexor digiti minimi brevis
Opponens digiti minimi

Execution

1. Sit on a bench with your feet flat on floor and grasp a bar with a closed, supinated grip, hands hip-width apart. Rest your elbows and forearms on top of your thighs with your wrists and hands anterior to—or in front of—the knees.
2. Raise the bar up as far as possible by flexing your wrists without moving your elbows or forearms.
3. Allow your wrists to slowly extend back to the starting position.

Muscles Involved

Primary: Flexor carpi radialis, palmaris longus, flexor carpi ulnaris

Secondary: Flexor digitorum superficialis, flexor digitorum profundus, opponens digiti minimi, flexor digiti minimi brevis

PREVENTIVE FOCUS

Wrist injuries typically occur with repetitive strain. Loading these structures helps to improve their strength, thereby reducing the likelihood of wrist muscle strain or wrist sprain. Because these muscles attach near the medial joint line of the elbow, it can also help reduce the risk of UCL injury.

When pitching a baseball, the ball must be gripped and manipulated in a variety of ways to produce the different types of pitches (e.g., fastball, change up, slider). This variety of grips and movements requires proper strength of the wrist flexors. In addition, the activity occurs at rapid velocities and is performed repeatedly. The combination of all these factors increases the likelihood of wrist flexor injury. By strengthening these muscles, their tolerance for high velocity, repetitive movements increases and the risk of injury decreases.

Wrist Roller

Fasten a weight to a dowel with a rope and allow the weight to hang down. Hold the dowel with a closed, pronated grip, hands 4 to 6 inches (10-15 cm) apart. With your arms at shoulder level, slowly roll the weight upward, curling your right hand over and down and then curling your left in the same way. Continue until the weight touches the dowel. Slowly reverse the motion and allow the weight to lower to the starting position.

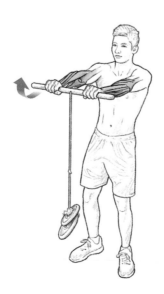

FOREARM SUPINATION AND PRONATION

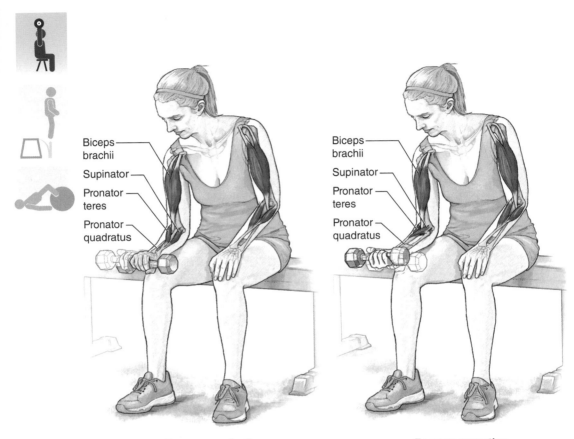

Biceps brachii

Supinator

Pronator teres

Pronator quadratus

Biceps brachii

Supinator

Pronator teres

Pronator quadratus

Forearm supination   **Forearm pronation**

Execution

1. Sit on a bench with your feet flat on the floor and grasp the middle (as shown) or the end of a dumbbell in your right hand with a closed, pronated grip, elbow flexed at 90 degrees. Rest your right elbow and forearm on top of your thigh with your wrist and hand anterior to—or in front of—the knees.

2. Turn the dumbbell up and over as far as possible by supinating your forearm without lifting your elbow or forearm.

3. Turn the dumbbell up and over as far as possible in the opposite direction by pronating your forearm without lifting your elbows or forearms.

4. Repeat with the left arm.

Muscles Involved

Primary: Biceps brachii, supinator, pronator teres

Secondary: Pronator quadratus

PREVENTIVE FOCUS

Many sports require a "turn of the wrist" (i.e., pronation or supination); this exercise helps to strengthen the muscles involved in such wrist movement as well as reduce the risk of UCL and wrist injuries.

The importance of wrist extension strength for tennis was discussed earlier in this chapter, but pronation also becomes important, especially when attempting to shape the shot. Although a forehand ground stroke does not inherently involve a lot of pronation, when the tennis player attempts to add topspin to the shot, the pronators become more involved. By strengthening these muscles, the tennis player is able to improve performance while also reducing injury risk.

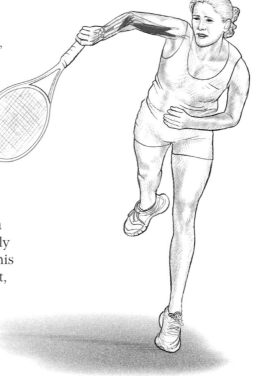

VARIATION

Forearm Supination and Pronation With Bat

Exchanging the dumbbell for a longer object—such as a bat—increases the resistance arm, thereby increasing the challenge and intensity of the exercise.

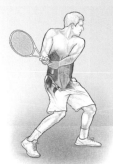

5

SPINE AND TRUNK

The spine and trunk are among the most commonly injured regions in both sport and daily life. Injuries to this region can be debilitating, with the potential to become chronic impediments to function. Reducing the risk of injuries to this area can appear daunting at first, but through a thoughtful examination of its structures, a blueprint for risk reduction emerges. Discussion of this region will be divided into the spine, including the vertebral column and the muscles and structures directly involved in its function, and the trunk, which comprises the other structures (primarily muscles) that help support the spine's movements.

SPINE

The function of the spine is to protect the spinal cord—a collection of nerves and pathways that carry signals between the brain and the rest of the body. The spine is made up of bones—vertebrae—and muscles and is traditionally divided into five sections—the cervical, thoracic, lumbar, sacral, and coccygeal (see figure 5.1)—each of which serves a unique function. The bones, most of which are separated by intervertebral discs, articulate with each other via facet joints and have openings between them that allow branches of the spinal cord to travel to different parts of the body as peripheral nerves. Each vertebra also has a posteriorly positioned spinous process, which offers some protection but primarily acts as an attachment point for muscles.

• *Cervical.* The top seven vertebrae in the spine, C1 to C7, connect to the base of the skull and are responsible for movement and normal functioning of the neck. The top two vertebrae—C1 and C2, commonly referred to as the *atlas* and *axis*—each have a unique structure, allowing for an articulating connection between the skull and the spine. Cervical injuries were detailed in chapter 3.

• *Thoracic.* The next 12 vertebrae, T1 to T12, serve as attachment points for the ribs.

• *Lumbar.* The lumbar vertebrae, L1 to L5 (also referred to as the low back), comprise the largest weightbearing area of the spine. This section of the spine is the most commonly injured and will be an area of focus for this chapter.

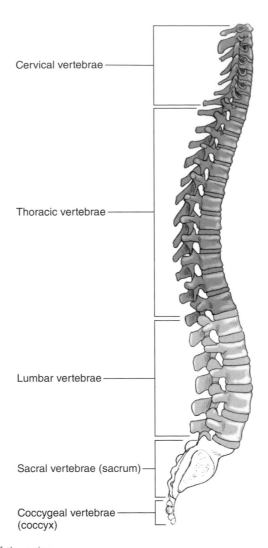

Cervical vertebrae

Thoracic vertebrae

Lumbar vertebrae

Sacral vertebrae (sacrum)

Coccygeal vertebrae
(coccyx)

FIGURE 5.1 Anatomy of the spine.

• *Sacrum.* The next five vertebrae, S1 to S5, provide the attachment between the spine and pelvis—the sacroiliac (SI) joint. All five of these vertebrae are fused together, with no discs between them, and the SI joint is stabilized by a collection of very stout ligaments. Although some movement occurs here, it is minimal; however, it can be a common location of pain.

• *Coccyx.* The lowest four vertebrae make up the coccyx; like the sacrum, these vertebrae are fused together. Injuries to this area of the spine are most commonly caused by falls.

Ligaments help to connect each vertebra to the next and therefore provide a significant amount of stability. When viewed from the side, the cervical and lumbar sections of the spine have lordotic curves, and the thoracic spine has a kyphotic curve (see figure 5.1). These spinal curves provide stability to help maintain balance while upright and support the weight of the head and upper body. Except in the fused sacrum and coccyx, intervertebral discs separate the vertebrae. These discs help to provide spacing for the peripheral nerves, as well as providing some cushioning. They allow the spine to bend and twist naturally. Each disc has two separate areas: The annulus fibrosus, comprised of tough collagen fibers, encircles the softer interior nucleus pulposus.

In addition to the ligaments and discs, the vertebral column is surrounded by muscles that stabilize and move the body. These muscles can be divided into superficial, intermediate, and deep muscles (see figure 5.2).

The superficial layer includes the splenius muscles—divided into cranial and cervical portions—which originate from the lower half of ligamentum nuchae, the lateral aspect of mastoid process, and the lateral third of the superior nuchal line (of the occipital bone of the skull). These muscles insert on the spinous processes of the upper six thoracic vertebrae (T1-T6) and the transverse processes of the upper four cervical vertebrae (C1-C4). When acting on one side only (i.e., unilaterally), they produce lateral flexion (commonly referred to as *side bending*) and rotation of the head and neck to the same side; when acting on both sides (i.e., bilaterally), they produce extension of the head and neck.

The intermediate layer is made up of the erector spinae muscles. This massive muscle group forms a bulge on either side of the vertebral column and is arranged in three vertical columns: iliocostalis (lateral column), longissimus (intermediate column), and spinalis (medial column). All erector spinae muscles

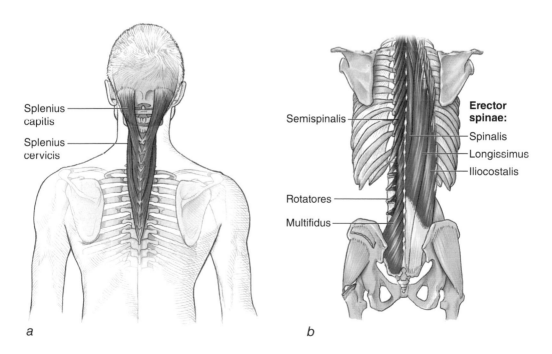

a　　　　　　　　　　　　　　*b*

FIGURE 5.2 *(a)* Superficial and *(b)* intermediate and deep muscle layers of the spine.

originate from the common erector spinae origin (a broad tendon attached to the posterior part of the iliac crest, the posterior sacrum, and the spinous processes of the sacrum and inferior lumbar spine) and insert throughout the lumbar, thoracic, and cervical spinous and transverse processes and the proximal region of the ribs. Acting bilaterally, erector spinae extends the head and part or all of the vertebral column; acting unilaterally, lateral flexion (side bending) of the head or vertebral column results.

The three deep muscles of the back are semispinalis, multifidus, and rotatores. In addition to movement and stability, these muscles stabilize the vertebral column and also help with balance and proprioception. These individual muscles originate on the transverse process of one vertebra and insert on the spinous process of a vertebra (or skull) one to two (rotatores), two to four (multifidus), or four to six (semispinalis) segments above the origin level.

The two most common types of back injuries involve either the muscles or intervertebral discs. Though fractures and ligamentous injuries do occur, they do not happen as often and may not be avoided through injury prevention exercises.

Lumbosacral Muscle Strain

Lumbosacral muscle strain—an injury of the paraspinal muscles in the low back—is one of the most common injuries to the low back (Will et al. 2018). As discussed in chapter 1, a strain is technically a tear of the muscle, graded as I, II, or III, depending on the degree of tearing, with the majority of lumbosacral muscle strains being microtears. These can be traumatic, but they can occur with gradual onset as well. The strain can result in pain and spasm, specifically in the involved muscles, although they can be diffused over a larger area as well. These symptoms tend to worsen with standing, lifting, and twisting motions. Despite common belief, there is limited evidence to suggest poor posture and improper lifting mechanics contribute to the risk of lumbosacral muscle strain.

Lumbar Disc Herniation

Lumbar disc herniation is a movement of disc material beyond its usual intervertebral disc space. This herniation process begins from failure in the ringed fibers of the annulus fibrosis, which causes an outward movement or bulging (typically in a posterolateral direction). When the bulge progresses to a great enough degree, the nucleus pulposus can push through the annular fibers; this is the herniation. Like lumbosacral muscle strains, lumbar disc herniations may develop traumatically or with gradual onset. The pain caused by disc herniation is likely a combination of nerve compression by the bulging disc and a local increase in inflammatory agents. Activity-related risk factors for disc injury are also not well understood at this time.

TRUNK

The trunk—also termed the *abdominal wall*—serves four primary functions:

- It protects the abdominal organs (e.g., liver).
- It is a repository for fat, especially for males.
- It aids in respiration.
- Its muscles produce movements of the vertebral column.

The surface anatomy of the trunk is unique and has three fibrous bands. The linea alba is a median fibrous white line or band joining the xiphoid process (of the sternum) to the pubic symphysis (joint between halves of the pelvis) and divides the anterior abdominal wall into right and left halves. This is seen on the surface of the abdomen as a vertical skin groove. The linea semilunaris is a curved line that extends from the ninth costal cartilage to near the pubic symphysis and both indicates the lateral border of rectus abdominis and separates rectus abdominis from external oblique muscles (see figure 5.3). The linea semilunaris is indicated by convex grooves 2 to 4 inches on either side of the linea alba. Tendinous inscriptions are horizontal lines on rectus abdominis.

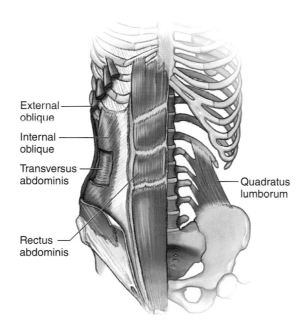

FIGURE 5.3 Abdominal and trunk muscles.

There are five muscles of the trunk: rectus abdominis, external oblique, internal oblique, transversus abdominis, and quadratus lumborum. Because of its role in spinal flexion and extension, erector spinae can be considered a trunk muscle as well.

• *Rectus abdominis.* This muscle originates on the pubic symphysis and the pubic crest and inserts on the xiphoid process (of the sternum) and costal cartilages 5 to 7. It flexes the trunk and is the primary flexor of lumbar vertebrae.

• *External oblique.* This muscle originates on the outer surfaces of ribs 5 to 12 (lower 8) and blends (interdigitates) with the serratus anterior insertion and the latissimus dorsi origin. External oblique inserts on the linea alba, the pubic tubercle, and the anterior half of the iliac crest. When acting bilaterally, it helps with flexion of the trunk; flexion and rotation of the trunk to the opposite side occur when they are acting separately. An easy way to remember the direction its muscle fibers are oriented is that the angle is similar to the direction one's fingers would be when inserting a hand into a front pocket.

• *Internal oblique.* Internal oblique is deep to external oblique and originates from the anterior two-thirds of the iliac crest and the lateral half of the inguinal ligament. It inserts on the inferior borders of ribs 10 to 12, the linea alba, and the pubis. Like external oblique, when these muscles act bilaterally, it helps with flexion of the trunk. When acting unilaterally, however, its actions are the opposite of external oblique; that is, they produce flexion and rotation of the trunk to the same side. Interestingly, internal oblique can produce flexion and rotation of the trunk to the opposite side when acting separately and with a fixed thorax.

• *Transversus abdominis.* The deepest of the abdominal muscles, transversus abdominis originates from the internal surfaces of costal cartilages 7 to 12 (lower six), the iliac crest, and the lateral third of inguinal ligament. It inserts on the linea alba (with internal oblique) and the pubic crest. Although it does assist with stabilization of the trunk, its primary role is compression and support of abdominal organs.

• *Quadratus lumborum.* This deep muscle originates from the inferior border of the 12th rib and the transverse processes of lumbar vertebrae; it inserts on the iliolumbar ligament and iliac crest. Quadratus lumborum helps to extend the vertebral column and its actions produce lateral flexion of vertebral column.

Injuries to the trunk generally involve the muscles to various degrees. The following two injuries described involve muscles either at one of their bony attachments or in the muscle belly itself.

Athletic Pubalgia

Athletic pubalgia, core muscle injury, or as it is often called, "sports hernia", is a strain or tear of any soft tissue in the lower abdomen or groin. The muscles most frequently affected by athletic pubalgia are the oblique muscles in the lower abdomen and the adductors of the thigh, primarily the muscle attachments to the pubic bone. Sporting activities that involve twisting under load can cause a tear in the soft tissue of the lower abdomen or groin. Athletic pubalgia occurs mainly in vigorous sports requiring rapid changes of direction, like football, soccer, and ice hockey. This injury usually results in pain in the groin area at the time of the injury. It can improve with rest, but often returns with a resumption of sporting activity, especially with twisting movements. Despite commonly being termed *sports hernia*, athletic pubalgia does not cause a visible bulge in the groin, like the more common inguinal hernia does.

Hip Pointer

A hip pointer is a deep bruise to the iliac crest, often due to a direct blow or fall, especially during contact sports (e.g., football, ice hockey) or those that involve falling on the side (e.g., volleyball, skateboarding). Those with a hip pointer typically describe pain and tenderness over the affected area. Recovery from the injury usually involves taking a break from activity until it heals.

DEADLIFT

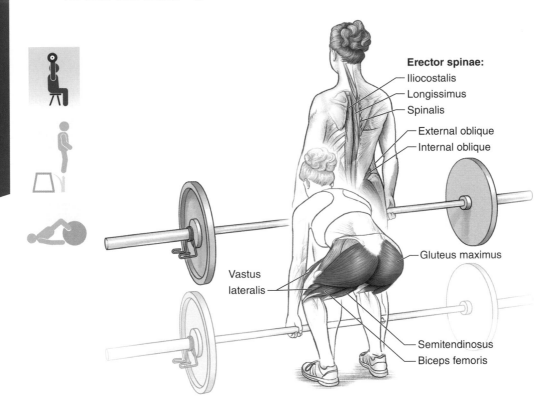

Erector spinae:
Iliocostalis
Longissimus
Spinalis
External oblique
Internal oblique
Gluteus maximus
Vastus lateralis
Semitendinosus
Biceps femoris

Execution

1. Stand with your feet flat on the floor shoulder- to hip-width apart and your toes pointed slightly outward.

2. Squat down and grasp the bar with a closed, pronated grip, hands shoulder-width apart.

3. *Note*: At this bottom position, your hips should be lower than your shoulders, the barbell should be approximately 1 inch (3 cm) in front of your shins, and your back should be flat with your chest held up and out.

4. Maintain a flat-back back position and keep your elbows straight as you lift the bar off the floor. Extend your hips and knees to produce this motion until you are standing straight up and down. Do not allow your hips to rise faster than your shoulders.

5. Still maintaining the flat-back back position, slowly lower the bar to floor by flexing your hips and knees.

Muscles Involved

Primary: Gluteus maximus, hamstrings (semitendinosus, semimembranosus, biceps femoris), quadriceps (rectus femoris, vastus lateralis, vastus medialis, vastus intermedius)

Secondary: Hip abductors, hip adductors (adductor longus, adductor magnus, adductor brevis), erector spinae (iliocostalis, longissimus, spinalis), rectus abdominis, external and internal obliques, transverse abdominis

PREVENTIVE FOCUS

The deadlift involves the use of all trunk and thigh muscles and, to be performed correctly, requires proper lower body and trunk alignment. Because of these factors, the deadlift is an excellent exercise to reduce the risk of spine and trunk injuries.

Most sporting activities benefit from incorporating the deadlift in an injury prevention program. Football linemen and cheerleading bases are two good examples of athletes who would derive particular benefit from the deadlift. The lineman must rise from a semisquat position against resistance, whereas the cheerleading base must support a fellow cheerleader. Strong muscles and good alignment reduce the risk of injury while performing these activities.

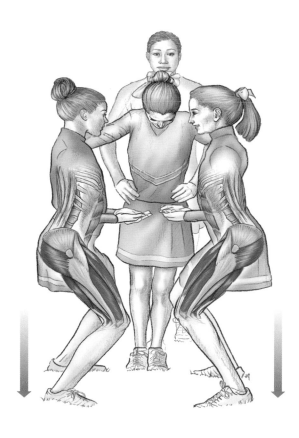

SIDE PLANK

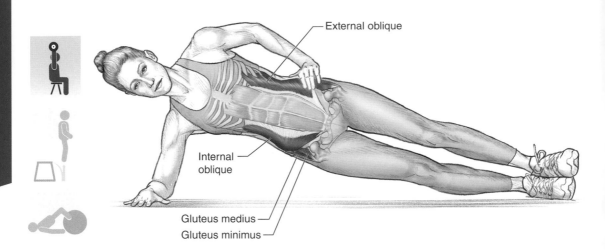

SPINE AND TRUNK

External oblique

Internal oblique

Gluteus medius

Gluteus minimus

Execution

1. Lie on the floor on your right side, with your right elbow beneath your right shoulder and right forearm perpendicular to your body.

2. Place your left foot on top of (or in front of) your right foot, rest your left hand on your hip, and hold your head in a neutral position, eyes focused forward.

3. Elevate your hips off the floor so the right ankle, knee, hip, and shoulder are in a straight line.

4. Isometrically hold the torso in a rigid position with your right elbow directly under your right shoulder, keeping your head in a neutral position.

Muscles Involved

Primary: External and internal obliques, gluteus medius, gluteus minimus

Secondary: Quadratus lumborum, erector spinae (iliocostalis, longissimus, spinalis)

PREVENTIVE FOCUS

Increasing the strength of the spine and trunk muscles reduces the risk of injury for sports requiring a stable spine, such as gymnastics. Gymnasts are required to resist lateral spine and trunk deviation while performing a wide variety of skills and holding different body positions, making the side plank an excellent exercise to both improve performance and reduce the risk of injury.

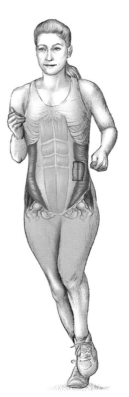

By increasing activation of the highlighted muscles, the side plank increases spinal stability and hip abductor strength. which has been shown to decrease injuries to those areas (Moffroid et al. 1993). Though the hip is more fully covered in chapter 6, it is important to mention the role of the side plank and hip abductor strength here. Several sports rely on the strength of this muscle to reduce injury risk. One such example is running: Every time a runner's foot hits the surface, the hip abductors must work eccentrically to resist hip adduction. By performing the side plank, runners can decrease the risk of hip and other lower extremity injuries.

VARIATION

Side Plank With Hip Abduction

Perform the side plank as described. When your hips are off the floor and your body is in a straight position, abduct the top lower extremity off the bottom lower extremity for the specified number of repetitions. Because the top lower extremity is no longer able to assist, this variation further challenges the hip abductors and trunk muscles.

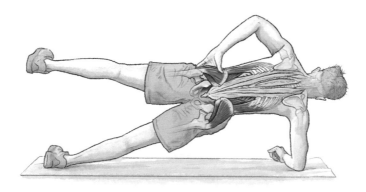

HALF-KNEELING PNF CHOP

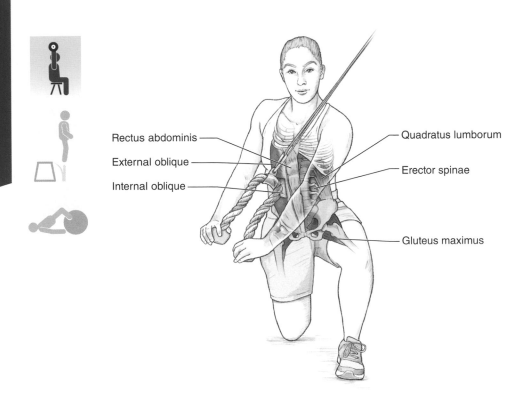

Rectus abdominis

External oblique

Internal oblique

Quadratus lumborum

Erector spinae

Gluteus maximus

Execution

1. Position yourself perpendicular to a cable machine and kneel on your outside leg with both knees bent at 90 degrees.
2. With a rope, handle, or bar, grab the weight from above with both hands and pull it down and across the body in a diagonal motion, from above the shoulder to the opposite hip, keeping the elbows extended.
3. Slowly return to the starting position.

Muscles Involved

Primary: Internal and external obliques, gluteus maximus

Secondary: Erector spinae (iliocostalis, longissimus, spinalis), rectus abdominis, quadratus lumborum

PREVENTIVE FOCUS

The half-kneeling PNF chop simulates the rotation movement that occurs in many sports, such as changing direction in football or soccer or defending in basketball. But one activity that especially benefits from this exercise is hitting a ball in baseball or softball. Hitting is a strong, rapid movement that requires the player to generate a significant amount of force and then just as quickly decelerate the motion caused from that force. Strengthening the muscles involved in this motion described helps to prepare them for activity and protect them from injury.

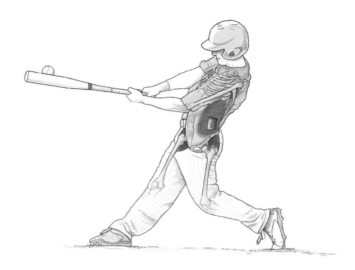

VARIATION

PNF Medicine Ball Chop

There are several variations of the half-kneeling PNF chop. This one is more ballistic and uses a medicine ball instead of a cable for resistance. To perform, assume the same half-kneeling position, but with the medicine ball held overhead. Bring your arms down and across toward your opposite hip and slam the ball into the floor.

STANDING PNF LIFT

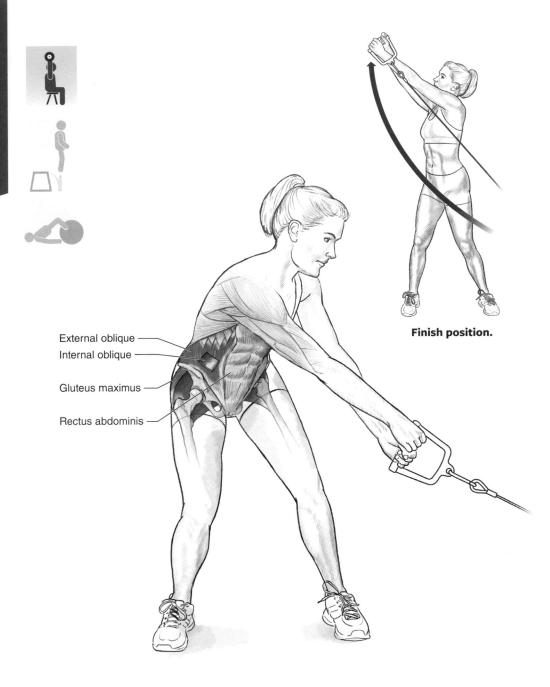

External oblique

Internal oblique

Gluteus maximus

Rectus abdominis

Finish position.

Execution

1. Stand perpendicular to a cable machine.
2. With a rope, handle, or bar, grab the weight from below with both hands and pull it up and across the body in a diagonal motion, from near the hip to above the opposite shoulder, keeping the elbows extended.
3. Slowly return to the starting position.

Muscles Involved

Primary: Internal and external obliques, gluteus maximus

Secondary: Erector spinae (iliocostalis, longissimus, spinalis), rectus abdominis, quadratus lumborum

PREVENTIVE FOCUS

Like the diagonal PNF chop, the standing PNF lift simulates the rotation that occurs in many sports, like hitting a tennis ball with a backhand stroke. Although commonly considered an upper extremity motion, the tennis backhand also involves muscles from the lower extremities and the trunk. If the focus is on the upper extremities only, the risk of spine or trunk injuries increases. By performing exercises that strengthen all the muscles required for tennis, the risk of those injuries decreases.

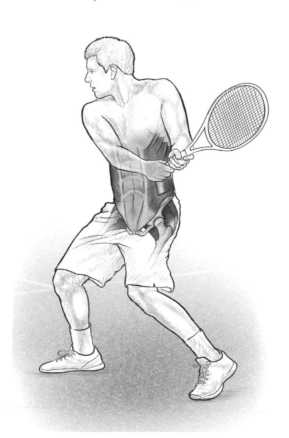

REVERSE HYPEREXTENSION

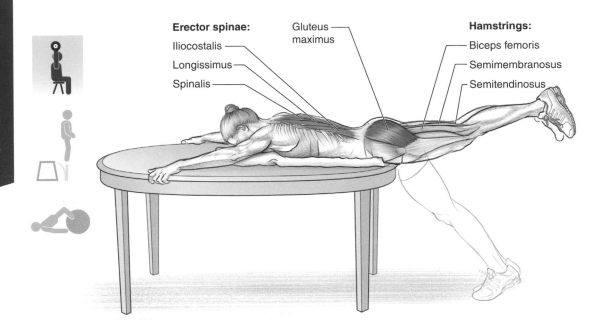

Execution

1. With your knees extended, assume a prone position on a table, hyperextension machine, or glute ham raise machine.
2. Hold onto the table with bilateral hands.
3. Keep the bilateral lower extremities together and lift at the same time until aligned with the trunk; avoid hyperextension of the lumbar spine.
4. Slowly lower to the starting position.

Muscles Involved

Primary: Erector spinae (iliocostalis, longissimus, spinalis), gluteus maximus

Secondary: Hamstrings (semitendinosus, semimembranosus, biceps femoris)

PREVENTIVE FOCUS

Strengthening the muscles of the back allows them to better stabilize the spine during sporting activity. This stability does not require the spine to not move, but rather for motion to occur in a relatively controlled manner. Swimmers are athletes that benefit from an exercise like the reverse hyperextension, especially when performing the freestyle and butterfly strokes. During these strokes, the spine extends and flexes (in addition to side bending and rotation). By strengthening the erector spinae muscles, they are better prepared for those motions, and the risk of spine and trunk injuries is thereby reduced.

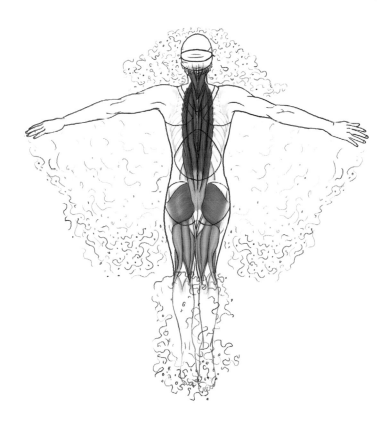

VARIATION

Medicine Ball Overhead Toss

This exercise variation simulates the explosiveness of many sports. Assume a comfortable, upright stance with your feet shoulder-width apart and hold a medicine ball at hip level. Lower the ball toward the floor and, using both arms, throw the ball up, back, and overhead to a partner.

MEDICINE BALL SIDE TOSS

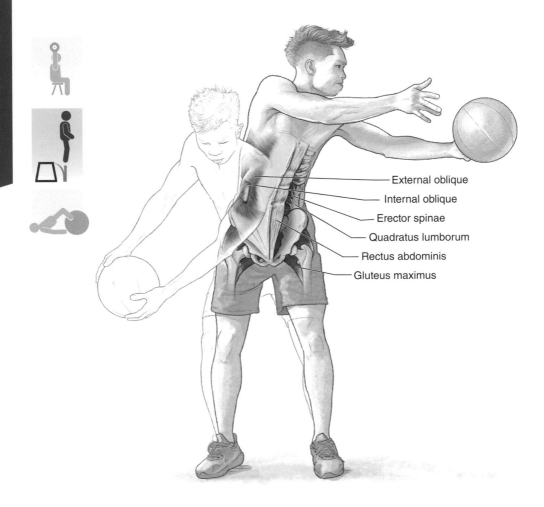

External oblique
Internal oblique
Erector spinae
Quadratus lumborum
Rectus abdominis
Gluteus maximus

Execution

1. Standing perpendicular to a wall approximately 6 feet (1.8 m) away, assume a comfortable, upright stance with feet shoulder-width apart, and hold a medicine ball at hip level.
2. Keeping your feet planted, turn your upper body away from the wall and throw the ball toward the wall using both arms.
3. Catch the ball as it rebounds and immediately repeat the throw.

Muscles Involved

Primary: Internal and external obliques, gluteus maximus

Secondary: Erector spinae (iliocostalis, longissimus, spinalis), rectus abdominis, quadratus lumborum

PREVENTIVE FOCUS

Strengthening the muscles that produce spine and trunk rotation helps to prepare these muscles for sporting activity. Like the half-kneeling PNF chop and standing PNF lift exercises, the side medicine ball toss simulates the rotation that occurs in many sports, like hitting a tennis ball or throwing a baseball or softball. Another example is the movement required by a football cornerback, who must backpedal and explosively turn and cover a receiver. The medicine ball side toss is an excellent exercise to prepare for this type of motion.

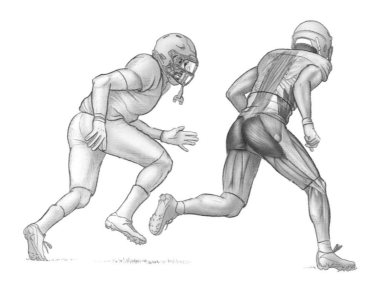

VARIATION

Shuffle to Side Toss

Begin this variation as with the medicine ball side toss; however, start the movement by shuffling two to three steps away from the wall. Plant the outside foot and throw the medicine ball into the wall, using both arms. The ball will likely drop to the floor; pick it up and repeat.

Note: Though not described in this chapter, two exercises require special mention: the Romanian deadlift (RDL) and Copenhagen hip adduction hold, both presented in chapter 7. Traditionally considered a hamstring exercise, the RDL also reduces the risk of low-back injuries. To properly perform this exercise, the athlete uses a mostly isometric contraction to target and overload the back extensors.

The Copenhagen hip adduction hold is an exercise used to reduce the risk of groin—or hip adductor muscle—injuries. This includes athletic pubalgia (as described in this chapter, athletic pubalgia can involve the hip adductor muscles).

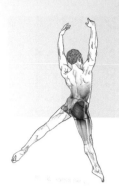

6

HIP

The hip is the joint between the pelvis and femur. The health and integrity of the hip joint is important for its own sake, but there is ample evidence that when the hip functions properly, other joints (specifically the knee and back) are better able to function as well. This chapter will review the relevant anatomy of the hip, its common injuries, and exercises to reduce the risk of those injuries.

The hip is a ball-and-socket joint that allows several degrees of movement. The combination of its bony structure and surrounding soft tissues results in a relatively stable joint with little required muscle activation.

The bones that make up the hip joint are the pelvis and the femur (see figure 6.1). The head of the femur (the ball) fits into the acetabulum (the socket). The acetabulum faces both anteriorly and laterally; the degree of forward or side orientation may predispose some to injury. The pelvis is formed by the ilium, ischium, and pubis bones. Like other joints, the articular surfaces of the pelvis and femur are covered with cartilage, but there is also a rim of cartilage that surrounds much of the socket. This rim is the acetabular labrum and is analogous to the glenoid labrum of the shoulder. Like its counterpart in the shoulder, the hip labrum can be torn or detached. Three primary ligaments join to form a capsule that surrounds the joint to provide further passive stability.

There are several muscles that surround the hip to both produce movement and to provide some additional stability. The muscles can be divided into posterior, anterior, and medial groups. Some of these muscles, including all of the medial muscles, are covered in chapter 7, when we discuss the thigh. Here, we take a closer look at the posterior and anterior muscles of the hip.

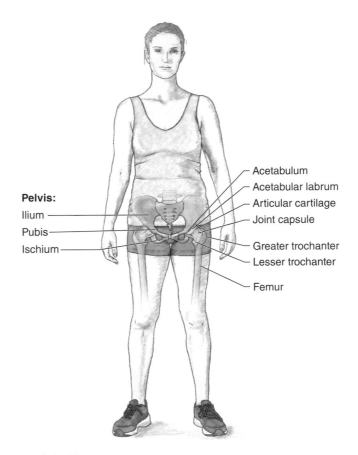

Pelvis:
Ilium
Pubis
Ischium

Acetabulum
Acetabular labrum
Articular cartilage
Joint capsule
Greater trochanter
Lesser trochanter
Femur

FIGURE 6.1   Anatomy of the hip.

POSTERIOR HIP MUSCLES

The posterior hip muscles can be divided into the larger, more superficial gluteals, and the deeper group of smaller muscles that are primarily responsible for lateral rotation of the thigh (see figure 6.2):

• *Gluteus maximus.* This is one of the strongest muscles in the body. When standing, gluteus maximus covers the ischial tuberosity; while seated (during hip flexion), the inferior border of the muscle slides superiorly, leaving the ischial tuberosity as a more superficial structure. The muscle originates from the iliac crest, sacrum, coccyx, and the sacrotuberous ligament. It inserts on the iliotibial band (IT band) and the gluteal tuberosity of the femur. Gluteus maximus is a powerful extender of the thigh at the hip joint; although it externally rotates the thigh as well, its main function is to bring the thigh from a flexed position into line with the body (e.g., when climbing stairs).

• *Gluteus medius.* This muscle is also on the posterior aspect of the hip. It is deep to gluteus maximus and has its origin on the external surface of the ilium, between anterior and posterior gluteal lines. It inserts on the lateral surface of the greater trochanter of the femur. Gluteus medius has three sections, which gives it the ability to perform multiple actions. This muscle abducts the thigh and performs both internal rotation (anterior portion) and external rotation (posterior portion) of the femur at the hip joint. It also helps to steady the pelvis when bearing weight on the same side (i.e., prevents the opposite side from dropping). In addition, gluteus medius helps to control inward (valgus) movement of the knee by limiting hip adduction and internal rotation when standing.

• *Gluteus minimus.* This is the deepest and smallest of the gluteal muscles. It originates from the external surface of the ilium, between anterior and inferior gluteal lines, and inserts on the anterior surface of the greater trochanter of the femur. It assists gluteus medius with abduction and internal rotation of the thigh at the hip joint.

• *Deep lateral rotators.* These six muscles are piriformis, obturator internus, superior gemellus, inferior gemellus, quadratus femoris, and obturator externus (although this muscle is anterior in position, it is functionally included with the lateral rotators). These muscles are commonly grouped because they have the same primary action and they generally function together. All six of these muscles have origins on the pelvis and insert on the greater trochanter. As their name indicates, they are responsible for laterally—or externally—rotating the thigh at the hip joint.

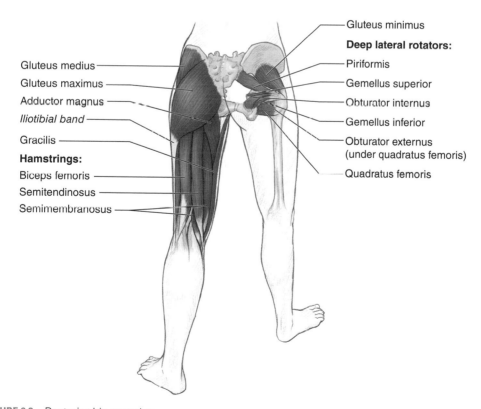

FIGURE 6.2   Posterior hip muscles.

ANTERIOR HIP MUSCLES

The anterior hip muscles have one primary purpose: to flex the thigh at the hip. Most are distinct structures, but some join together or insert with other muscles at common locations (see figure 6.3).

- *Iliopsoas.* Iliopsoas is made up of two muscles with unique origins that join at the same insertion point and perform same actions. Its primary function is flexion of the thigh at the hip joint, but it also provides some stability to the hip joint and can flex the trunk.
   - › *Psoas major.* This muscle originates on the sides of T12 to L5 vertebrae and intervertebral discs between them, and it inserts on the lesser trochanter of the femur.
   - › *Iliacus.* Originating on the iliac crest, iliac fossa, and anterior sacroiliac ligaments, iliacus inserts with psoas major on the lesser trochanter.
- *Tensor fasciae latae.* This small muscle originates on the anterior superior iliac spine (ASIS) and part of iliac crest; it inserts on the iliotibial (IT) band. This muscle assists with flexion, abduction, and medial rotation of the thigh at the hip joint, but it also has the unique action of tensioning the IT band and fasciae latae (a band of connective tissue that surrounds the thigh muscles), which enables the thigh muscles to act with increased force. Interestingly, because gluteus maximus also inserts on the IT band, tensor fasciae latae allows the gluteus maximus to assist in keeping the knee joint in the extended position.
- *Sartorius.* So named because of its unique pathway (sartorius crosses the thigh in the tailor's squatting position), this muscle originates primarily on the ASIS and inserts on the superior part of notch inferior to it (the notch formed by the ASIS and the anterior inferior iliac spine) and inserts on the superior part of medial surface of tibia. This insertion point—common with gracilis and semitendinosus—is referred to as the *pes anserinus* (mentioned in chapter 7).

ILIOTIBIAL BAND

One other structure must be mentioned as it is implicated in many injuries, the IT band. The IT band is a thick, fibrous tissue of fascia that runs distally from the iliac crest on the pelvis and has several insertions on the lateral proximal tibia (i.e., Gerdy's Tubercle and others). The IT band stabilizes the hip, especially in the frontal plane, and also stores a great amount of energy when running (Hutchinson et al 2022). When this energy is stored, it is released which improves running economy.

Hip pain and injury is a common cause of dysfunction for athletes. In the past, most hip pain was assumed to be a muscle-related injury. Although muscle can be a source of pain, our knowledge and understanding of the hip has revealed many other injuries as well. Common injuries of the hip may occur to the bony structures, muscles, tendons, and ligaments. Each type of injury has a unique mechanism and will be covered in the paragraphs that follow.

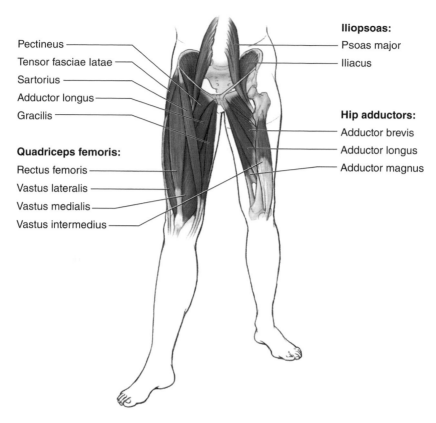

Iliopsoas:
- Psoas major
- Iliacus

Pectineus

Tensor fasciae latae

Sartorius

Adductor longus

Gracilis

Hip adductors:
- Adductor brevis
- Adductor longus
- Adductor magnus

Quadriceps femoris:

Rectus femoris

Vastus lateralis

Vastus medialis

Vastus intermedius

FIGURE 6.3   Anterior hip muscles.

Femoroacetabular Impingement (FAI)

Femoroacetabular impingement (FAI) involves either extra bone growth along the femoral head, atypical orientation of the acetabulum (the cup of the hip), or a combination of the two. This results in an irregular interface to the joint, which may result in the bones rubbing against each other during movement. Eventually, this contact may cause irritation or damage to the structures in the hip, causing pain and limiting activity. There are three types of FAI: pincer, cam, and combined. Pincer occurs because of a more downward or lateral orientation of the acetabulum, resulting in the bone of the anterior wall extending out over the typical rim location of the acetabulum. Cam occurs when additional bone grows out of the anterior junction of the femur, resulting in increased anterior joint compression during flexion and internal rotation of the hip. Combined impingement means that both the pincer and cam types are present. The cause of FAI morphology is unknown at this time and likely includes both hereditary and environmental factors. The presence of FAI without pain or dysfunction should be considered a normal presentation, specifically in athletes who present with a higher incidence. When painful, the pain primarily occurs in the front of the hip joint and down through the groin area. Turning, twisting, and deep squatting motions may increase the athlete's pain when symptomatic.

Greater Trochanteric Pain Syndrome

Greater trochanteric pain syndrome—sometimes referred to as *trochanteric bursitis* or *gluteal tendinopathy*—results from degenerative changes affecting the gluteal tendons and bursa. Bursae are small, fluid-filled sacs that often lie under (deep to) tendons to reduce friction. Athletes will report pain over the outside (lateral) aspect of the hip region that increases with impact-related activity like running, jumping, and landing. Those with weak hip abductors tend to experience greater hip adduction during activity, although it is unknown if this results in or is the result of pain. This increased adduction can result in compression of the gluteus medius and gluteus minimis tendons at the greater trochanter, which may add to the irritation of those tendons. Further, when hip adduction increases, the IT band can likewise exert greater compressive forces on the gluteal tendons. In sports, this increased hip adduction is often seen by a pelvic drop on the opposite side (see figure 6.4).

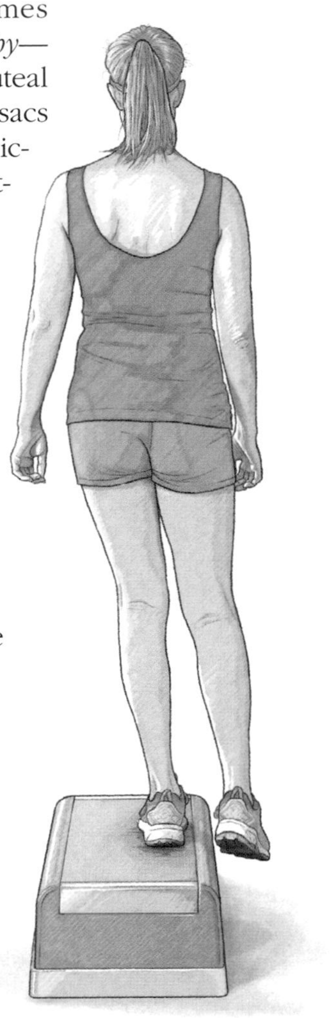

FIGURE 6.4 An example of pelvic drop.

Snapping Hip Syndrome

As its name indicates, snapping hip syndrome is a snapping sensation that can occur on the lateral, posterior, or anterior aspects of the hip. It typically occurs when forcefully lifting or swinging the lower extremity and involves the IT band or gluteus tendons sliding over the greater trochanter. Though not as common, posterior snapping involves one of the hamstring muscles rolling over the ischial tuberosity. Snapping at the anterior aspect of the hip can involve the iliopsoas tendon rolling over several structures—like bony prominences and even another part of the tendon—surrounding the hip, primarily near the front of the hip joint.

Hip Flexor Strain

There are several hip flexor muscles, but the most likely to become strained are the iliopsoas (iliacus and psoas major) and rectus femoris. This chapter will focus on iliopsoas strain; refer to chapter 7 for discussion of rectus femoris strain. Although both chronic and acute hip flexor strain exist, chronic is the more common of the two. Chronic, overuse injuries may result from any activity requiring repetitive, forceful hip flexion, like kicking a ball or sprinting. *Dancer's hip* and *jumper's hip* are variations of hip flexor strain that typically occur with repetitive hip flexion in an externally rotated position. Strains to the iliopsoas may have associated tendon irritation and anterior snapping. Acute injuries typically follow forceful eccentric contraction of the muscles or brisk flexion against an external force (e.g., the playing surface or an opponent) that surpasses the capacity of the tendon.

IT Band Syndrome

IT band syndrome is an overuse injury and is common in runners and cyclists. The IT band has been implicated in snapping hip (discussed earlier) and as a friction-related injury. It has been proposed that the IT band rubs over the lateral femoral condyle causing friction which leads to pain. However, recent research indicates compression—not friction—actually occurs at this interface between the lateral femoral condyle and the IT band irritating the nerves deep to the IT band (Archbold and Mezzadri 2014; Fairclough et al. 2007). This is important as it is likely not caused from being too tight as is commonly thought (Fairclough et al. 2007; Hutchinson et al. 2022). However, the cause of IT band syndrome remains unclear.

SIDE-LYING HIP ABDUCTION

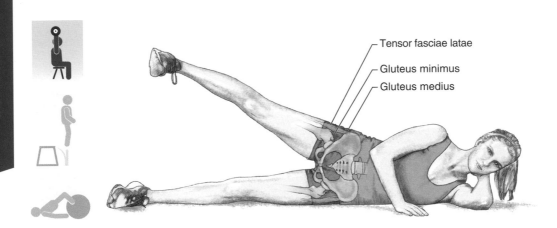

- Tensor fasciae latae
- Gluteus minimus
- Gluteus medius

Execution

1. Lie on your side with one lower extremity resting on top of the other and your feet pointed straight ahead.
2. Keeping your knees straight, point your top foot slightly downward, and lift your top lower extremity 6 to 8 inches (15-20 cm) without moving the foot forward.
3. Slowly lower to the starting position.
4. *Note:* The intensity of this exercise can be increased by adding a cuff weight or other external resistance to the top lower extremity.

Muscles Involved

Primary: Gluteus medius, gluteus minimus

Secondary: Tensor fasciae latae

PREVENTIVE FOCUS

Strengthening the hip abductors not only improves their strength and function, it also improves the function and reduces the risk of knee injury (Stearns-Reider et al. 2021). Although the clamshell exercise is commonly used for this purpose, the side-lying hip abduction is more effective at recruiting the hip abductor muscles (Moore et al. 2020).

As briefly mentioned in chapter 5, the hip abductors play an important role in activities such as running by working to reduce hip adduction when the athlete's foot strikes the ground. This is especially important in basketball because hip adduction leads to a dynamic valgus movement, a risk factor for knee injury—especially ACL tear, which is very common in basketball.

Although the strength of other muscles is important, strong hip abductors reduce the risk of ACL and other knee injuries by resisting the hip adduction portion of dynamic valgus movements.

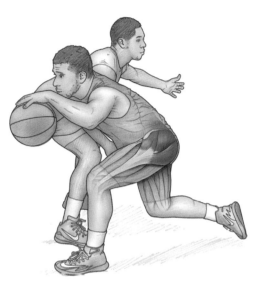

VARIATION

Wall Isometric Hip Abduction

As its name indicates, this exercise involves an isometric contraction of the hip abductors, but instead of just one side, both hip abductors are involved. To perform, stand to one side of a wall or door frame. Standing on one foot, flex the hip closest to the wall to 90 degrees and place the outside (lateral aspect) of the knee against the wall. From this position, push the outside of the knee into the wall; hold for a prescribed time and repeat on both sides. The abductors of the flexed hip are actively pushing the outside of the knee into the wall while the abductors of the other hip are isometrically active to maintain hip and pelvis alignment.

MANUAL ECCENTRIC HIP ABDUCTION

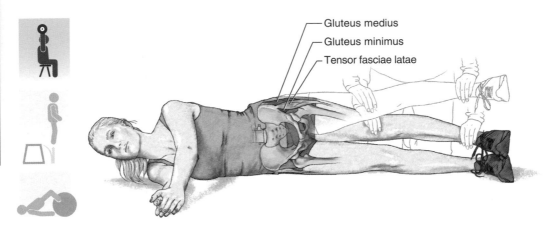

Gluteus medius
Gluteus minimus
Tensor fasciae latae

Execution

1. Lie on your side with a partner kneeling behind.
2. Keeping your knee straight, lift the top lower extremity approximately 12 inches (30 cm) above the bottom lower extremity.
3. Have your partner place one hand just above the knee of your top lower extremity and the other hand on your ankle and push the top leg down toward the bottom lower extremity. Resist this motion as much as you are able.
4. Once your top lower extremity touches your bottom lower extremity, raise it again and repeat the exercise.

Muscles Involved

Primary: Gluteus medius, gluteus minimus

Secondary: Tensor fasciae latae

PREVENTIVE FOCUS

As stated previously, strengthening the hip abductors—especially in an eccentric manner—not only improves their strength and function, it also improves the function and reduces the risk of knee injury (Stearns-Reider et al. 2021), especially for athletes in sports involving running and those requiring deceleration with a single lower extremity. As discussed with running previously, when the foot strikes the ground, the hip tends to adduct; the hip abductors act eccentrically to slow this motion and reduce this inward movement. One of the common mechanisms of IT band friction syndrome, a frequent injury among cross-country runners, is the hip adduction described here. An exercise like eccentric hip abduction decreases hip adduction and therefore reduces the risk of IT band friction syndrome.

Any athlete who must land on a single lower extremity, such as a ballet dancer, would also benefit from eccentric hip abduction. When landing from a leap, the dancer must stabilize the weightbearing lower extremity. As with cross-country running, the hip abductors act eccentrically to help provide this stability. Hip injuries are quite common in ballet; stronger hip abductors (the goal of this exercise) reduces the risk of these injuries.

VARIATIONS

Closed Chain Eccentric Hip Abduction

Another way to work on eccentric hip abduction is in a closed chain. To do this, stand on a step with your right foot while the left foot is off the step. Keeping your right knee straight, lower your left hip toward the floor, then lift up as high as you are able. The majority of the motion for this exercise should be coming from the hip, with a small degree coming from the spine. This exercise involves the hip abductors of the lower extremity standing on the step—in this case, the right side.

Resisted Side Step

A popular exercise to strengthen the hip abductors is a resisted side step, sometimes referred to as a *monster walk*. Start by standing with a resistance band around your ankles and your feet turned in. Keeping your knees extended, step to the right with your right foot, then slowly allow the left foot to step to the right, maintaining tension in the band throughout the exercise. Repeat for a given distance (e.g., 30 feet), then return to the starting position leading with the left foot.

BENCH BRIDGE OR HIP THRUST

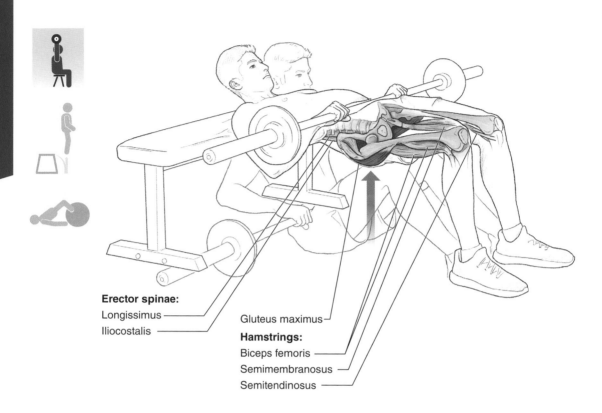

Erector spinae:
Longissimus
Iliocostalis

Gluteus maximus
Hamstrings:
Biceps femoris
Semimembranosus
Semitendinosus

Execution

1. Sitting on a bench with both feet on the floor, hold a barbell across your waist with both hands.
2. Step your feet forward until only your shoulder blades are in contact with the bench, still keeping both feet on the floor.
3. Begin the exercise with your knees, hips, and shoulders in a straight line.
4. Keeping your shoulder blades on the bench, lower (flex) the hips toward the floor.
5. Lift your hips to return to the starting position.

Muscles Involved

Primary: Gluteus maximus

Secondary: Hamstrings (semitendinosus, semimembranosus, biceps femoris), erector spinae (iliocostalis, longissimus, spinalis)

PREVENTIVE FOCUS

Strengthening the hip extensors prepares these muscles for sporting motions, but doing so also helps to provide stability to both the hip and knee joints. Because the gluteus maximus externally rotates the thigh and inserts on the IT band, it helps to stabilize the knee during hip extension. Further, when the gluteus maximus provides hip extension, it does not need to rely as heavily upon the hamstrings to assist with this motion. Because hamstring use during the hip extension phase of sprinting has been implicated as a possible hamstring injury mechanism, strengthening the gluteal muscles can reduce the risk of injury for sprinters.

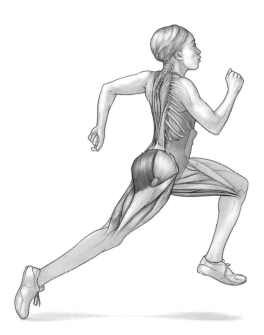

VARIATION

Single-Leg Bench Bridge

One progression of the bench bridge is to perform the exercise with a single foot in contact with the floor. To do this, simply lift one foot off the floor and perform the exercise as previously described. This is a more challenging variation of the bench bridge and requires the muscles of the lower extremity in contact with the floor to control and produce the required movement. As with many exercises, adding increased external resistance, like a barbell or medicine ball, is yet another way to progress.

FORWARD LUNGE

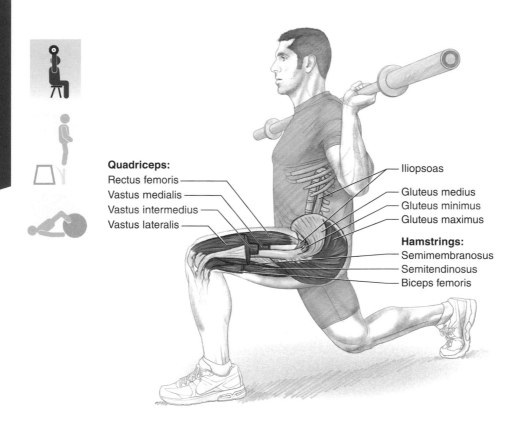

Quadriceps:
Rectus femoris
Vastus medialis
Vastus intermedius
Vastus lateralis

Iliopsoas
Gluteus medius
Gluteus minimus
Gluteus maximus

Hamstrings:
Semimembranosus
Semitendinosus
Biceps femoris

Execution

1. Place a barbell behind your head and across your shoulders and take one exaggerated step directly forward with one lower extremity, keeping your torso erect.

2. Plant the lead foot flat on the floor pointing straight ahead, allowing the trailing knee to slightly flex.

3. Once balance has shifted to be even on both feet, allow your lead hip and knee to slowly flex and your trailing knee to lower toward the floor. Your lead knee should be aligned with the second and third toes of the lead foot (which remains flat on the floor).

4. Lower your trailing knee—still slightly flexed—until it is 1 to 2 inches (3-5 cm) above the floor. At this point, your lead knee will be flexed to about 90 degrees, with the lower leg perpendicular to the floor (actual lunge depth depends primarily on individual hip joint flexibility).

5. Balance your weight evenly between the ball of the trailing foot and the entire lead foot.

6. Shift your balance forward to the lead foot, and forcefully push off the floor to return to the starting position by extending your lead hip and knee, still maintaining the same torso position.

Muscles Involved

Primary: Gluteus maximus, hamstrings (semitendinosus, semimembranosus, biceps femoris), quadriceps (rectus femoris, vastus lateralis, vastus medialis, vastus intermedius)

Secondary: Iliopsoas, gluteus medius, gluteus minimus

PREVENTIVE FOCUS

The forward lunge has many benefits: Not only are the identified muscles strengthened, but proper lower extremity (primarily knee) alignment is reinforced. The lunge is especially beneficial for athletes who rely on deceleration and quick direction changes, like soccer players. When approaching an opponent with the ball, an offensive player often plants a foot, pushes off that foot, and then changes direction. This sudden deceleration is the action most likely to lead to injury and may be performed more safely if deceleration strength on a single lower extremity is a focus during training. The forward lunge is an excellent introduction to that type of training.

VARIATION

Side Lunge

This exercise is performed with the same steps as the forward lunge, but to the side. Place a barbell behind your head and across your shoulders and perform an exaggerated step to the left with your left foot. With your foot pointing straight ahead, flex your left knee and lower your body to a comfortable depth. Maintain proper knee alignment (i.e., knee lined up with second and third toes). The trailing (right) knee remains extended during the side lunge. Forcefully push off and return the left foot to the starting position.

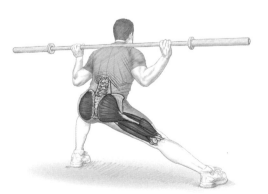

SPLIT SQUAT JUMP

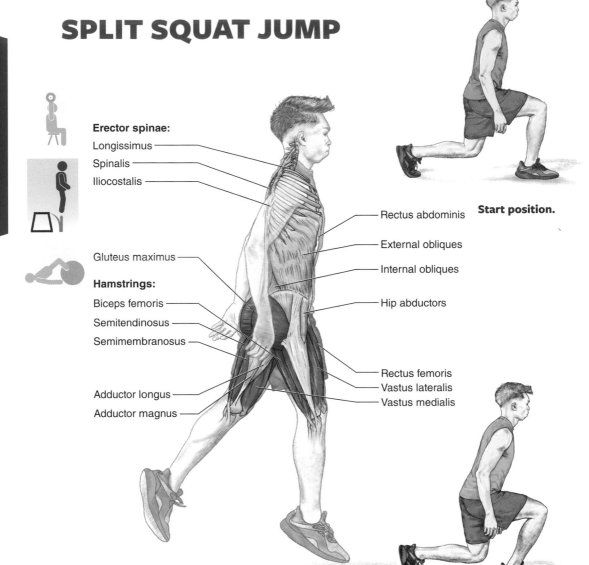

Erector spinae:
Longissimus
Spinalis
Iliocostalis

Rectus abdominis

External obliques

Internal obliques

Gluteus maximus

Hamstrings:

Biceps femoris

Semitendinosus

Semimembranosus

Hip abductors

Adductor longus

Adductor magnus

Rectus femoris
Vastus lateralis
Vastus medialis

Start position.

Finish position.

Execution

1. Stand in a split squat position with one lower extremity forward and the other behind your body. Both the hip and knee joints should be flexed to approximately 90 degrees.

2. Maintaining proper knee alignment with the lead lower extremity, squat down slightly and immediately jump up, using both arms to assist.

3. When landing, maintain the same split squat position and immediately repeat the jump. Focus on proper knee alignment and maximum jump height.

Muscles Involved

Primary: Gluteus maximus, hamstrings (semitendinosus, semimembranosus, biceps femoris), quadriceps (rectus femoris, vastus lateralis, vastus medialis, vastus intermedius)

Secondary: Hip abductors, hip adductors (adductor longus, adductor magnus, adductor brevis), erector spinae (iliocostalis, longissimus, spinalis), rectus abdominis, external and internal obliques, transverse abdominis

PREVENTIVE FOCUS

The split squat jump is a good plyometric exercise to work on both explosiveness and knee alignment. The front lower extremity is challenged to avoid dynamic valgus movement and jumping from this squat position is challenging for the involved muscles, especially those on both the anterior and posterior aspects of the hips.

• *Anterior.* Though the activity of the front lower extremity is responsible for much of the work performed, the anterior aspect of the back lower extremity undergoes a stretch at the bottom position and assists in the jump. In addition, when preparing to land, the back lower extremity undergoes a rapid eccentric muscle contraction, which is similar to the movement in many sporting activities.

• *Posterior.* The front lower extremity is responsible for the majority of the work performed during this exercise. In addition, at the bottom position, the muscles of the posterior hip are stretched maximally; these same muscles are then responsible for helping the athlete jump in the air. As with the anterior muscles, the posterior muscles undergo a rapid eccentric muscle contraction when landing.

Sprinting and soccer are two of the most common examples of sports that involve this rapid eccentric to concentric actions of the hip flexors. The split squat jump helps to replicate that rapid motion.

VARIATION

Cycled Split Squat Jump

The cycled split squat jump is very similar to the split squat jump and begins the same way, but while in the air, switch your front and back lower extremities so that upon landing, their positions are reversed. As with the split squat jump, sprinters and soccer players benefit from performing this exercise: Both sprinting as well as long passes and shots involve the hip flexors transitioning from eccentric to concentric contractions.

7

THIGH

Although it is not defined by a specific joint or series of joints, the thigh—the area between the hip and knee—has unique, commonly injured structures that necessitate a detailed discussion (see figure 7.1). Most injuries to the thigh occur in the soft tissue, particularly the muscle. Although the bone of the thigh (femur) and nerves within the thigh can suffer injuries, these are much less common than injuries to the structures that surround them.

The muscles of the thigh are commonly divided into three compartments: anterior, posterior, and medial. Because there is a significant crossover of muscles between the thigh and the adjacent hip and knee joints, especially the hip, some muscles are covered in chapters 6 and 8.

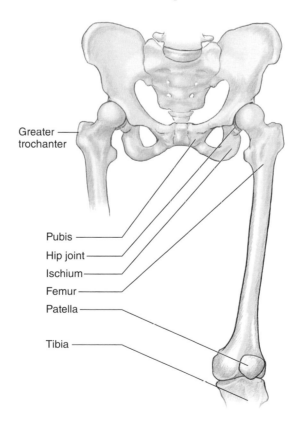

Greater trochanter

Pubis

Hip joint

Ischium

Femur

Patella

Tibia

FIGURE 7.1 Anatomy of the thigh and upper leg.

ANTERIOR THIGH

The anterior thigh has one large group of muscles (quadriceps femoris) as well as four others (psoas major, iliacus, tensor fasciae latae, and sartorius), which are covered in chapter 6 on hip injury prevention. Quadriceps femoris (referred to as simply quadriceps going forward), as its name indicates, is composed of four individual muscles: rectus femoris, vastus lateralis, vastus medialis, and vastus intermedius (see figure 7.2). As they join together, all four of these muscles have a common insertion: the patellar base and tibial tuberosity via the patellar tendon.

• *Rectus femoris.* This muscle originates from the anterior inferior iliac spine and works with the other quadriceps muscles to extend the leg at the knee joint. Because its origin is proximal to the hip joint and therefore crosses that joint, it assists the combined iliopsoas muscle with hip stabilization and flexion of the thigh at the hip joint. This is the only quadriceps muscle to perform these actions at the hip and is the only quadriceps muscle not to have a direct connection with the femur.

• *Vastus lateralis.* This muscle originates on the lateral aspect of the femur, specifically the greater trochanter and lateral lip of the linea aspera of the femur. It works with the other quadriceps muscles to extend the leg at the knee joint.

• *Vastus medialis.* This muscle also originates on the thigh, but as its name indicates, it originates on the medial aspect of the femur, specifically the intertrochanteric line and medial lip of the linea aspera of the femur. It works with the other quadriceps muscles to extend the leg at the knee joint.

• *Vastus intermedius.* The fourth quadriceps femoris muscle lies between vastus lateralis and vastus medialis and originates on the anterior and lateral surfaces of the femur. It works with the other quadriceps muscles to extend the leg at the knee joint.

As indicated, these muscles unite to form the quadriceps tendon, which attaches to the patellar base and surrounds the patella, then continues as the patellar tendon to attach to the tibial tuberosity. Of note, though the connection between the patella and tibial tuberosity may be termed a ligament (because it connects two bones together), it is commonly referred to as a tendon. Functionally, ligaments stabilize joints and tendons help muscles pull on bones to produce motion. Because the quadriceps muscle force pulls on the tibial tuberosity to produce knee extension, it functions as a tendon, not a stabilizing ligament.

As mentioned previously, injuries to bones and nerves are possible, but most injuries that occur in the anterior aspect of the thigh are muscular in nature. These muscles are required to perform two primary jobs, deceleration and acceleration. These roles require rapid eccentric and concentric muscle actions, respectively.

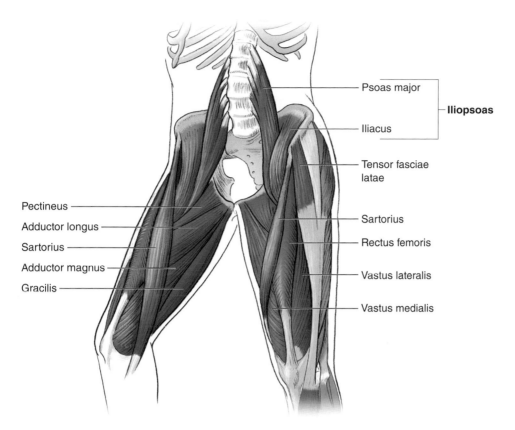

FIGURE 7.2   Anterior thigh muscles.

Quadriceps Strain

A quadriceps muscle strain usually follows an acute tearing of one or more of the quadriceps muscles and is common in sports requiring repeated sprinting, quick changes of direction, and frequent decelerations, like soccer and basketball. Though there are four muscles that constitute the quadriceps femoris complex, the three vastii muscles (vastus lateralis, vastus medialis, and vastus intermedius) are the ones affected here; rectus femoris will be covered in the next section. Quadriceps strain is similar to but must be differentiated from two other injuries to the anterior thigh:

- *Muscle cramp* is a micro spasm to the muscle belly.
- *Muscle contusion* is a deep bruise to the quadriceps muscles following a direct blow or trauma.

Though most quadriceps strains are acute in nature, overuse injuries can occur. Acute strains can occur following rapid movements like sprinting, kicking, and changes of direction, whereas overuse injuries often follow activities involving repeated eccentric activity of the quadriceps, like running downhill.

Rectus Femoris Strain

Strain of the rectus femoris muscle is the tearing of those muscle fibers. Because of this muscle's unique two-joint arrangement (it attaches above the hip on the anterior inferior iliac spine and below the knee on the tibial tuberosity) and actions (hip flexion and knee extension), the mechanism is similar to that of both quadriceps strain and hip flexor strain—that is, the knee is flexed and hip is extended. Typically, athletes participating in sports that involve sprinting and kicking are more likely than others to strain this portion of the quadriceps muscle complex.

MEDIAL THIGH

The medial (inner) compartment of the thigh is made up of five muscles with similar functions: adduction of the thigh at the hip and stabilization during stance (see figure 7.2). A sixth medial thigh muscle, obturator externus, is addressed with the gluteal muscles in chapter 6.

• *Pectineus.* This muscle originates from the pectineal line of the pubis, lateral to the pubic tubercle, and inserts on the pectineal line of the femur. It adducts the thigh at the hip joint and assists with flexion of the thigh, also at the hip joint.

• *Adductor longus.* This is the most anterior adductor muscle and originates from the body of the pubis, inferior to the pubic crest. It inserts on the middle third of linea aspera of the femur and adducts the thigh at the hip joint.

• *Adductor brevis.* This muscle lies deep to pectineus and adductor longus and anterior to adductor magnus. It originates on the body and inferior ramus of the pubis and inserts on the pectineal line and proximal part of the linea aspera of the femur. Although its main function is adduction of the thigh at the hip joint, it assists with flexion as well.

• *Adductor magnus.* The largest of the adductor muscles, adductor magnus has two portions, the adductor and hamstring parts. This muscle originates from the inferior ramus of the pubis and the ramus of the ischium (adductor part) and the ischial tuberosity (hamstring part). The adductor part inserts on the gluteal tuberosity, linea aspera, and supracondylar line of the femur; the hamstring part inserts on the adductor tubercle of the femur. Adductor magnus is responsible for adduction of the thigh, flexion of the thigh (adductor part), and extension of the thigh at the hip joint (hamstring part).

• *Gracilis.* This is the most superficial of the adductor muscles and therefore it is the most medial muscle of the thigh. It originates from the body and inferior ramus of the pubis and inserts on the superior part of the medial surface of the tibia, along with two other muscles of the hip and thigh (sartorius and semitendinosus) join to form a common fanlike insertion into the tibia, *pes anserinus.* (Because of its appearance, it was thought to look like the foot of a goose, hence the name: pes = foot; anserinus = goose.) Gracilis adducts the thigh at the hip joint and, because it crosses the knee joint, assists with flexion of the leg at the knee joint. Of all the adductor muscles, it generates the least amount of force. Because of this, gracilis can be removed without noticeable loss of function and is often used by surgeons as a graft to repair a damaged muscle or to reconstruct other structures, like the ACL.

Like the hamstring muscles, the adductor muscle group plays multiple roles in sporting activity. This combination of stability and assisting with changes of direction places the muscles at an increased risk of injury.

Adductor Strain

A strain of the hip adductors (colloquially referred to as *groin pull* or *strain*) produces pain when pressing on the hip adductor tendons and their insertion on the pubic bone. Typically, these injuries also result in pain with resisted hip adduction. This injury typically occurs during sports requiring twisting, sprinting, kicking, or changes of direction, like ice hockey, soccer, and football.

POSTERIOR THIGH

The three large muscles in the posterior compartment of the thigh, collectively termed the *hamstring muscles*, are the semitendinosus, semimembranosus, and biceps femoris (see figure 7.3). The hamstrings have a common origin at the ischial tuberosity and span both the hip and knee joints. Because of this, the hamstrings act at both joints (though not at the same time).

• *Semitendinosus.* This muscle inserts on the superior part of the medial surface of the tibia, the pes anserinus. Semitendinosus extends the thigh at the hip joint and flexes the leg at the knee joint. This hamstring muscle lies medially to biceps femoris and, along with biceps femoris, lies superficially (nearer the surface) to the other musculature of the posterior compartment.

• *Semimembranosus.* This hamstring muscle lies deep to both semitendinosus and biceps femoris and, like semitendinosus, lies in the medial half of the posterior compartment. It inserts on the posterior part of the medial condyle of the tibia and has the same action as semitendinosus (extension of the thigh at the hip joint and flexion of the leg at the knee joint).

• *Biceps femoris.* Although the primary actions of biceps femoris are the same as semitendinosus and semimembranosus, this hamstring muscle differs from the other two hamstrings in that it has two sections—or heads—and inserts on a different bone. The long head originates from the ischial tuberosity with the other hamstring muscles, whereas the short head originates from the femur (lateral lip of the linea aspera and the lateral supracondylar line). Both heads join to insert on the lateral side of the fibular head; this is different from the tibial insertion of the other hamstring muscles. Along with semitendinosus, the long head of biceps femoris lies superiorly to other musculature of the posterior compartment, and the short head of biceps femoris lies deep to both the long head of biceps femoris and semitendinosus; both heads lie laterally to semitendinosus.

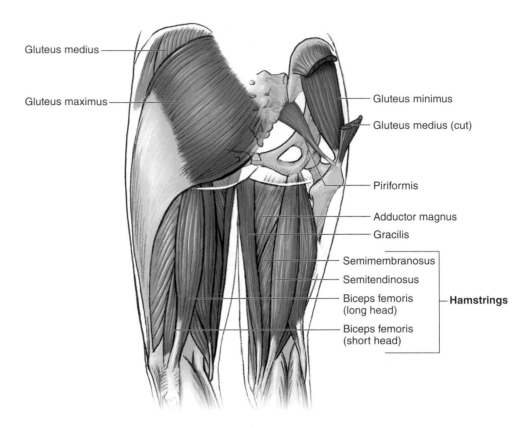

FIGURE 7.3   Posterior thigh muscles.

The anatomy and function of the hamstring muscles predispose them to injury. Being a two-joint muscle group requires the muscles to act at both the hip and knee joints. This can cause challenges of active or passive insufficiency—that is, the muscles become too short or too long (respectively) to generate force. In addition to the bony attachments, the hamstrings perform multiple roles, especially when running at high speeds. The hamstrings must slow the forward motion of the lower extremity through an eccentric muscle contraction and then immediately generate concentric force to rapidly move the lower extremity. This combination of unique architecture and dual function creates challenges that can lead to injury if not properly trained.

Hamstring Strain

Hamstring injuries are one of the most common noncontact injuries in sports like football, soccer, rugby, and sprinting (Brooks et al. 2006; Drezner et al. 2005; Ekstrand et al. 2010; Feeley et al. 2008). Like other muscle strains, hamstring muscle strains may be grade I, II, or III, depending on the degree of tearing. Of the three hamstring muscles, biceps femoris is the most commonly injured, with the musculotendinous junction and adjacent muscle fibers being the most common injury sites. The cause of hamstring strains is complex, and like many injuries, involves multiple factors. In the previously mentioned sports, hamstring injury rates range from 10 to 26 percent of all injuries sustained (Drezner et al. 2005); further, recurrence rates are even higher—up to 32 percent (Heiser et al. 1984). There are many risk factors for hamstring injury, but the most common are older age, previous hamstring injury, history of ACL injury, and previous calf strain injury (Green et al. 2020). Reduced hamstring strength is also related to an increase in the risk of hamstring injury (Freckleton et al. 2014; Goossens et al. 2015; Schuermans et al. 2016). Perhaps surprisingly, there is little—if any—research to support the notion that decreased hamstring flexibility is a risk factor for hamstring strain (Green et al. 2020).

Reducing the risk of hamstring injury has traditionally focused on several areas, including strength, flexibility, and endurance. In recent years, the focus has shifted to eccentric exercises (van Dyk et al. 2019), strengthening in lengthened positions (Marušič 2020), strengthening both hip- and knee-biased motions (Bourne et al. 2017), and sprinting (Higashihara et al. 2018; Mendi-guchia et al. 2020). We advocate a combination of these approaches to most efficiently reduce the risk of hamstring injuries and an example of each focus is provided in this chapter.

Sprinting for Injury Prevention

Sprinting has recently been examined as an exercise mode to reduce injury risk (Prince et al. 2021). Sprinting is a key part of many sports and relies on significant hamstring contribution to perform most effectively. In other words, greater horizontal ground reaction force results in greater the sprinting speed. The hamstrings—specifically biceps femoris—significantly contribute to this increased horizontal ground reaction force. Sprinting also requires the hamstrings to be very active during swing and just prior to ground contact in order to decelerate the quickly advancing lower extremity. This combination of concentric (propulsion of mass) and eccentric (deceleration of lower extremity) forces is unique and, unless properly trained, may be lacking. One area of exploration has been fascicle length of biceps femoris. Fascicle length is basically the length of a group of muscle fibers. This is important as greater fascicle length has been associated with improved sprinting performance (Kumagai et al. 2000) and reduced risk of injury. Both the Nordic hamstring curl (found later in this chapter) and sprinting increase fascicle length of biceps femoris, though sprinting is able to do this in a moderately improved way. The fascicle length change and its importance in injury prevention is likely due to an improved force–length relationship of the hamstrings through an increase of in-series sarcomeres (Proske and Morgan 2001) and increases in tendon stiffness (Butterfield and Herzog 2005). Therefore, including sprinting in an injury prevention program is quite important (Morin 2015).

BACK SQUAT

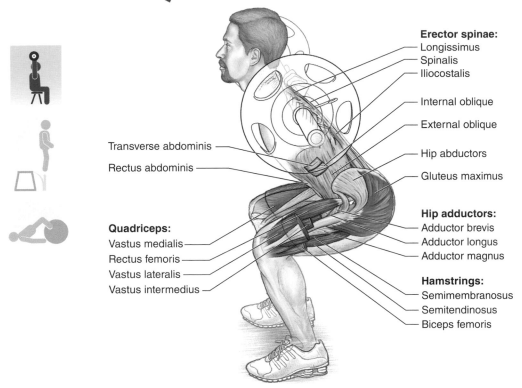

Erector spinae:
Longissimus
Spinalis
Iliocostalis

Internal oblique

External oblique

Hip abductors

Gluteus maximus

Hip adductors:
Adductor brevis
Adductor longus
Adductor magnus

Hamstrings:
Semimembranosus
Semitendinosus
Biceps femoris

Transverse abdominis

Rectus abdominis

Quadriceps:
Vastus medialis
Rectus femoris
Vastus lateralis
Vastus intermedius

Execution

1. Step under the rack and place your hands on the barbell in a closed, pronated grip.
2. Holding your chest up and out, lift your elbows to create a shelf for the bar to rest across your back.
3. Extend your hips and knees to lift the bar off the rack, and take one or two steps backward, keeping your elbows lifted up to keep the bar on your shoulders.
4. Position your feet shoulder-width apart or wider with your toes slightly pointed outward.
5. Allow your hips and knees to slowly flex while keeping the torso-to-floor angle constant.
6. *Note*: Maintain a flat-back position with your elbows high and your chest up and out. Keep your heels on the floor and your knees aligned with the second and third toes of the feet.

7. Continue allowing your hips and knees to flex until your thighs are parallel to the floor.

8. Extend your hips and knees, still keeping the torso-to-floor angle constant.

9. *Note*: Continue to maintain a flat-back position with your elbows high and your chest up and out. Keep your heels on the floor and your knees aligned with the second and third toes of the foot.

10. Continue extending the hips and knees to reach the starting position.

11. After the set is completed, step forward and rack the bar.

Muscles Involved

Primary: Gluteus maximus, hamstrings (semitendinosus, semimembranosus, biceps femoris), quadriceps (rectus femoris, vastus lateralis, vastus medialis, vastus intermedius)

Secondary: Hip abductors, hip adductors (adductor longus, adductor magnus, adductor brevis), erector spinae (iliocostalis, longissimus, spinalis), rectus abdominis, external and internal obliques, transverse abdominis

PREVENTIVE FOCUS

The back squat involves the use of all the thigh muscles and, to be performed correctly, requires proper lower body and trunk alignment. Improper alignment has been implicated in many injuries, including knee injuries (see chapter 8).

Because it requires the use of so many muscles and can help with deceleration, jumping, and reinforcing lower extremity alignment, the back squat has applications for nearly all sports involving the lower extremities. Volleyball is an excellent example of a sport whose players would particularly benefit from incorporating the back squat into training, because every position on the floor uses the squatting motion during matches:

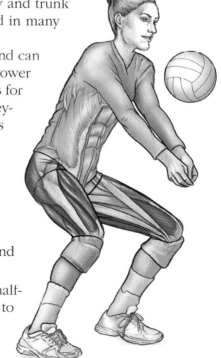

- When landing from a jump, blockers should squat down, even if only slightly.

- When landing from a hit, outside hitters absorb the landing impact by bending their knees and squatting.

- Defensive specialists are often positioned in half- to three-quarter squat position in preparation to receive the ball from the opposing team.

- Setters squat and jump up during the jump set.

(continued)

BACK SQUAT *(continued)*

VARIATIONS

Slant Board Squat

The slant board squat increases muscle activity of the quadriceps (and other structures) to a greater degree than the standard back squat (Kongsgaard et al. 2006). Specifically, the increased eccentric stress increases the strength of those muscles, especially when used during deceleration motions. Stand toward the bottom of a slant board so your heels are toward the top of the board with both feet pointing down, and perform the standard back squat. This exercise is typically performed without weight to start but can be added as you progress. At the lowest point of the squat, the knees should be in front of the toes. Squatting with the back and heels against a wall will force proper form if needed.

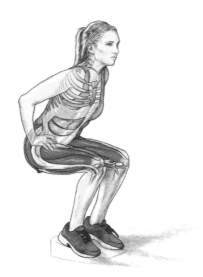

Single-Leg Squat

The single-leg squat is essentially the same exercise as the back squat but performed on one leg versus two. There are several variations of the single-leg squat (e.g., pistol squat, Bulgarian split squat, skater's squat). More detail on the single-leg squat is provided in chapter 8.

SINGLE-LEG PUSH-OFF

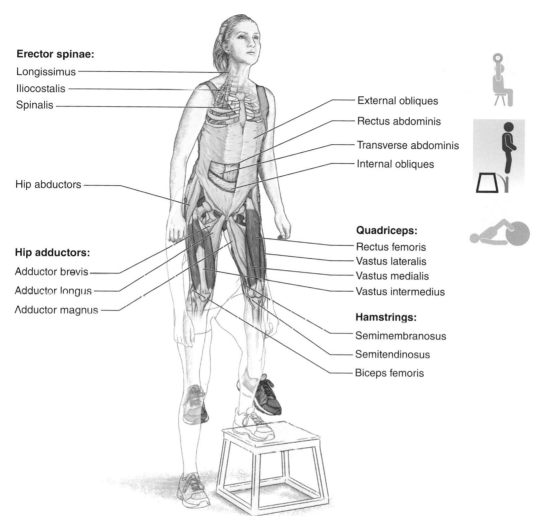

Erector spinae:
Longissimus
Iliocostalis
Spinalis

External obliques

Rectus abdominis

Transverse abdominis

Internal obliques

Hip abductors

Quadriceps:
Rectus femoris
Vastus lateralis
Vastus medialis
Vastus intermedius

Hip adductors:
Adductor brevis
Adductor longus
Adductor magnus

Hamstrings:
Semimembranosus
Semitendinosus
Biceps femoris

Execution

1. Stand next to a plyometric box with one foot on the ground and one foot on the box.

2. Using the foot on the box to push off, jump in the air, focusing on proper knee alignment.

3. Land with the same foot on the box and allow your other foot to touch the floor; the foot on the box should land just before the foot on the ground.

4. Immediately repeat the jump.

(continued)

SINGLE-LEG PUSH-OFF *(continued)*

5. *Note:* Intensity may be increased by increasing the height of the box. Begin with a height of 6 inches (15 cm); boxes up to 18 inches (45 cm) high may be used, depending on the athlete's height (taller athletes require taller boxes).

Muscles Involved

Primary: Gluteus maximus, hamstrings (semitendinosus, semimembranosus, biceps femoris), quadriceps (rectus femoris, vastus lateralis, vastus medialis, vastus intermedius)

Secondary: Hip abductors, hip adductors (adductor longus, adductor magnus, adductor brevis), erector spinae (iliocostalis, longissimus, spinalis), rectus abdominis, external and internal obliques, transverse abdominis

PREVENTIVE FOCUS

The focus of this exercise helps to reinforce lower extremity alignment when jumping and landing on a single limb. Because the athlete begins with the knee and hip in flexed positions, the involved muscles are more stretched than when jumping from the floor. This requires greater muscle activity than standard plyometric exercises because the amortization phase is longer than it is for other continuous or countermovement jumps. The continuous nature also helps to simulate the movements common in sporting activities. This exercise is appropriate for all sports that require athletes to jump and land on a single leg, such as figure skating. Although the surface is different, all figure skating jumps require similar hip and knee positions as the single-leg push-off, making this exercise good preparation from both a strength and alignment standpoint.

VARIATION

Front Single-Leg Push-Off

In addition to changing the height of the box, you can change the focus of the exercise by facing the box instead of standing to the side. Although the quadriceps remain active, this variation tends to challenge the hamstrings and gluteal muscles to a greater degree than the standard single-leg push-off exercise, making it useful for hamstring injury prevention programs.

REVERSE BENCH BRIDGE

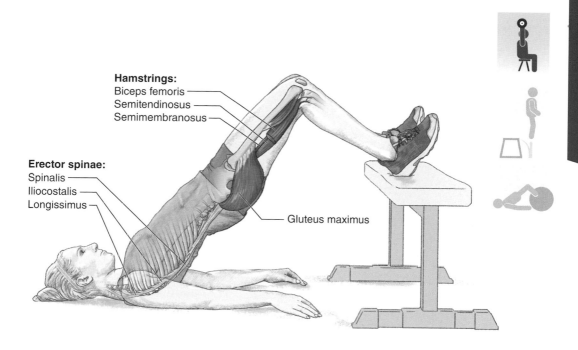

Hamstrings:
Biceps femoris
Semitendinosus
Semimembranosus

Erector spinae:
Spinalis
Iliocostalis
Longissimus

Gluteus maximus

Execution

1. Place a bench on the floor and lie supine, perpendicular to the bench with your knees straight and lower extremities parallel; your feet should be closest to the bench.

2. Keeping your hips on the floor and flexing your knees to 90 degrees, position the back of your heels on the bench.

3. Without moving your upper body, extend your hips until your knees, hips, and shoulders are in a straight line.

4. Allow your hips to lower and return to the starting position.

Muscles Involved

Primary: Hamstrings (semitendinosus, semimembranosus, biceps femoris), gluteus maximus

Secondary: Erector spinae (iliocostalis, longissimus, spinalis)

(continued)

REVERSE BENCH BRIDGE   *(continued)*

PREVENTIVE FOCUS

Because the hamstrings perform actions at both the hip and the knee, many exercises have a specific focus on one joint versus the other. The reverse bench bridge focuses on the hamstrings' function at the hip joint—specifically, thigh extension. The reverse bench bridge improves the ability of both the hamstrings and the gluteus maximus to function at the hip joint while also strengthening the hamstrings' attachment to the ischial tuberosity.

Athletes from several sports can benefit from strengthening the hamstrings in this manner. Sprinters, for example, rely on their hamstrings to help increase their speed when running. All exercises in this section will benefit sprinters, but the reverse bench bridge is particularly beneficial because it also engages gluteus maximus. Although research has yet to substantiate the common belief that hamstring strain can result because the gluteus maximus is not properly working, performing an exercise that uses both the hamstrings and gluteus maximus is beneficial to improve the function of both muscles during sprinting activities.

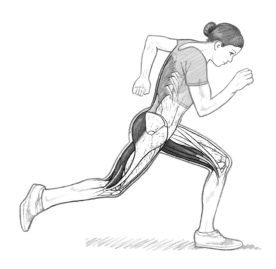

VARIATION

Plyometric Reverse Bench Bridge

Assuming the same starting position as the reverse bench bridge, rapidly extend the hips by driving upward. This motion should cause the feet to leave the bench. Land with the feet on the bench and lower the hips. Immediately repeat.

NORDIC HAMSTRING CURL

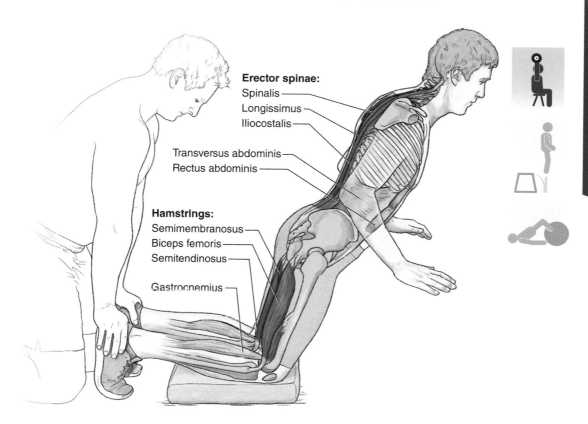

Erector spinae:
Spinalis
Longissimus
Iliocostalis

Transversus abdominis
Rectus abdominis

Hamstrings:
Semimembranosus
Biceps femoris
Semitendinosus

Gastrocnemius

Execution

1. Kneel on a soft surface on the floor (e.g., foam pad) with your knees flexed to 90 degrees and your knees, hips, and shoulders in a straight line.
2. Have a partner grasp your feet and ankles and hold them down.
3. Maintaining the same straight line through the knees, hips, and shoulders, slowly extend your knees and lower your torso forward to the floor.
4. *Note:* If you are unable to control the downward movement of your torso, allow yourself to fall, catching yourself with your hands.
5. Once your torso is on the floor, lift back to the starting position, still keeping your knees, hips, and shoulders in line.
6. *Note:* If you are unable to independently return to the starting position, use your arms to assist by pushing upward.

(continued)

NORDIC HAMSTRING CURL   *(continued)*

Muscles Involved

Primary: Erector spinae (iliocostalis, longissimus, spinalis), hamstrings (semitendinosus, semimembranosus, biceps femoris)

Secondary: Gastrocnemius, transversus abdominis, rectus abdominis

PREVENTIVE FOCUS

The Nordic hamstring curl involves a strong eccentric contraction of the hamstrings during the downward movement phase, which strengthens the muscles and reduces the risk of strain. By using this exercise, hamstring injury rates decrease by up to 70 percent (Al Attar et al. 2017; van der Horst et al. 2014; van Dyk et al. 2019); this dramatic impact is important to emphasize. Rarely does the addition of a single exercise reduce the risk of injury by such a great degree.

As with other hamstring-focused exercises listed in this chapter, the Nordic hamstring curl benefits any athletes that regularly sprint during practices or games. Baseball is an example that may not seem obvious at first, but hamstring injury rates for baseball players have steadily increased since 2011 (Okoroha et al. 2019). The most common mechanism is base running, specifically to first base. By incorporating the Nordic hamstring curl into training sessions throughout the year, the rate of hamstring injuries for these athletes should decrease.

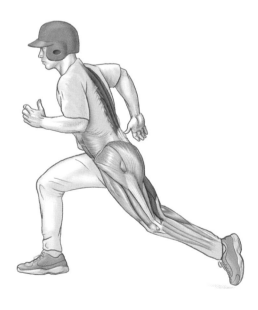

VARIATIONS

Harop Curl

The Harop curl involves the same motion as the Nordic hamstring curl, but instead of the downward and upward motion occurring at the knee joints, it occurs at the hip joint. Begin in the same starting position as the Nordic hamstring curl, but lower your torso toward the floor by allowing the hips to flex, and return to the starting position by extending your hips. This variation, though still relying on the hamstring muscles, also relies on gluteus maximus.

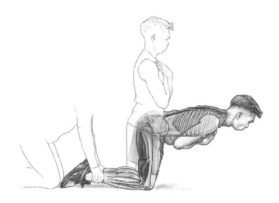

Razor Curl

Like the Harop curl, the razor curl has similar motions as the Nordic hamstring curl. Begin with your knees on the floor and both your hips and knees extended (as in the bottom position of the Nordic hamstring curl). Lift yourself up to 90 degrees of hip flexion and 90 degrees of knee flexion, then maintain 90 degrees of hip flexion while your knees continue to flex (Oliver and Dougherty 2009). Finally, return to the starting position.

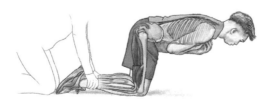

ROMANIAN DEADLIFT

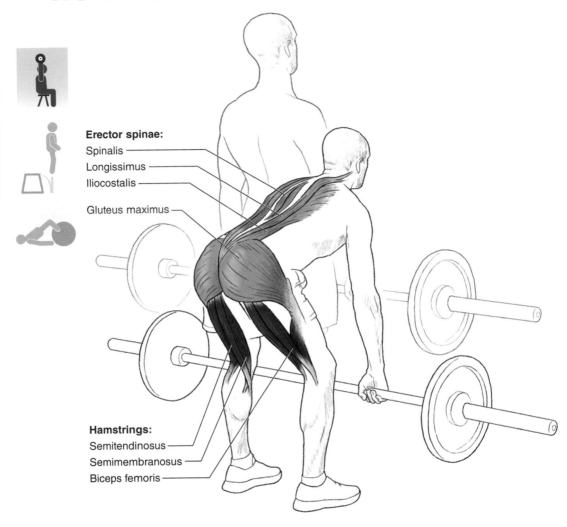

Erector spinae:
Spinalis
Longissimus
Iliocostalis

Gluteus maximus

Hamstrings:
Semitendinosus
Semimembranosus
Biceps femoris

Execution

1. Place your hands on the bar in a closed, pronated grip.
2. Lift the bar off the floor and slightly flex your knees (approximately 30 degrees); maintain this position throughout the exercise.
3. *Note*: All repetitions begin from this position.
4. Flex your hips and push them backward, allowing your torso to move forward and keeping the bar in contact with your thighs.
5. Maintaining the slightly flexed knee position and keeping your torso rigid with a neutral spine, lower until a stretch is felt in the posterior thigh (hamstrings).
6. Extend your hips and raise your torso to the starting position.
7. *Note*: Maintain the slightly flexed knee and neutral spine positions.

Muscles Involved

Primary: Hamstrings (semitendinosus, semimembranosus, biceps femoris)

Secondary: Gluteus maximus, erector spinae

PREVENTIVE FOCUS

Like the Nordic hamstring curl, the Romanian deadlift (RDL) involves a significant eccentric muscle action during the downward movement phase. The RDL, however, more closely mimics the actions of the lower extremities during the sprint motion; this specificity helps to strengthen the hamstrings in a sport-specific manner. Further, because of the stretch caused by the forward motion at the hips, the RDL helps to strengthen the hamstrings in a lengthened position.

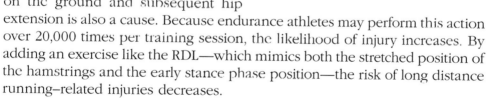

Although sprinting is a very common injury mechanism for hamstring injuries, running for prolonged periods (e.g., soccer games, long distance running) has also been shown to contribute to hamstring muscle strains (Jones et al. 2015). Although a hamstring strain can be stretch-induced (e.g., in the transition between the late swing and early stance phase), it is likely that the contact of the foot on the ground and subsequent hip extension is also a cause. Because endurance athletes may perform this action over 20,000 times per training session, the likelihood of injury increases. By adding an exercise like the RDL—which mimics both the stretched position of the hamstrings and the early stance phase position—the risk of long distance running–related injuries decreases.

VARIATION

Single-Leg Romanian Deadlift

The single-leg Romanian deadlift is similar to the Romanian deadlift, but is performed while balancing on one leg. This allows the athlete to improve balance while also making the movement more sport specific, because most sporting movements are performed on one leg at a time.

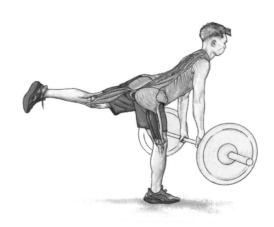

PIKE JUMP

POSTERIOR THIGH

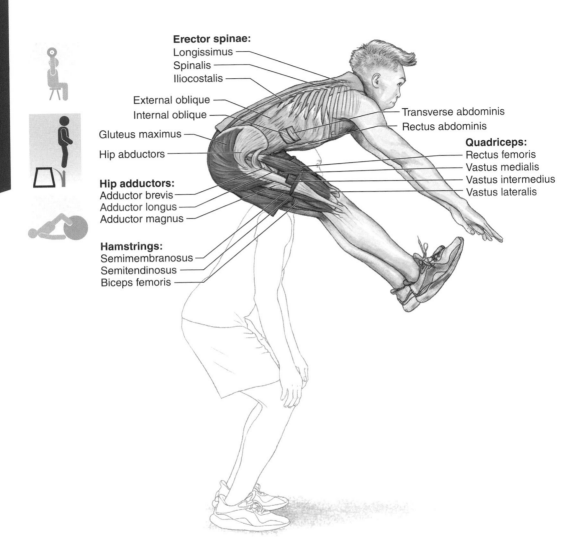

Erector spinae:
Longissimus
Spinalis
Iliocostalis

External oblique
Internal oblique

Gluteus maximus

Hip abductors

Hip adductors:
Adductor brevis
Adductor longus
Adductor magnus

Hamstrings:
Semimembranosus
Semitendinosus
Biceps femoris

Transverse abdominis
Rectus abdominis

Quadriceps:
Rectus femoris
Vastus medialis
Vastus intermedius
Vastus lateralis

Execution

1. Stand with your feet shoulder- to hip-width apart.
2. Keeping your knees in proper alignment, bend your knees slightly and jump in the air.
3. Keep your legs straight and together and lift them to the front (in a pike position) to touch your toes with your hands.
4. Land and immediately repeat the jump.

Muscles Involved

Primary: Gluteus maximus, hamstrings (semitendinosus, semimembranosus, biceps femoris), quadriceps (rectus femoris, vastus lateralis, vastus medialis, vastus intermedius)

Secondary: Hip abductors, hip adductors (adductor longus, adductor magnus, adductor brevis), erector spinae (iliocostalis, longissimus, spinalis), rectus abdominis, external and internal obliques, transverse abdominis

PREVENTIVE FOCUS

Like other plyometric exercises, the pike jump helps improve explosiveness. This exercise is unique for a variety of reasons—specifically, it requires rapid movement and hamstring flexibility to perform. It is this last point that makes the pike jump especially important for hamstring injury prevention programs. During this exercise, the athlete's hamstrings undergo a rapid stretch near their end range of flexibility at both the hip and the knee; then rapidly extend to allow the athlete to land on her feet. By undergoing this quick stretch, the hamstrings are better able to tolerate this motion and the risk of injury decreases.

Several sports require this movement, but dancers, cheerleaders, and gymnasts would particularly benefit from the pike jump because they require both flexibility and strength at the end range of hamstring motion.

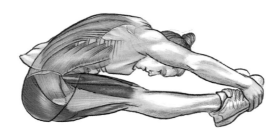

HIP FLEXOR HOLD

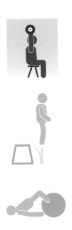

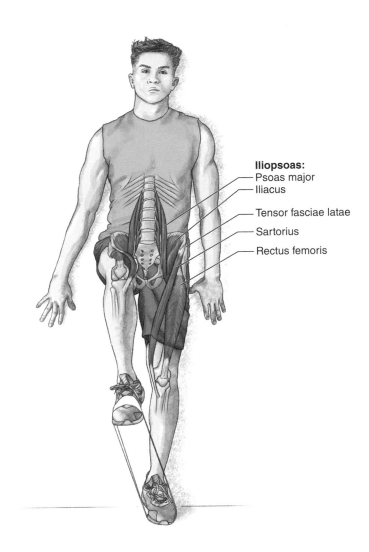

Iliopsoas:
Psoas major
Iliacus

Tensor fasciae latae

Sartorius

Rectus femoris

Execution

1. Stand with your back against the wall and an elastic loop placed around both feet.

2. Maintaining contact with the wall, flex your hip to lift your thigh until the top of the thigh is parallel with the floor.

3. Hold for the prescribed duration (e.g., 10 seconds), then slowly lower your thigh to the starting position.

Muscles Involved

Primary: Iliopsoas, rectus femoris, sartorius

Secondary: Tensor fasciae latae

PREVENTIVE FOCUS

Isometric muscle actions can produce greater muscle force than concentric muscle actions. By maintaining that force for a prolonged time, both strength (due to the isometric muscle action) and muscular endurance (due to the prolonged hold) of the hip flexors are increased. All athletes who perform sprinting activities would benefit from including this exercise in their training.

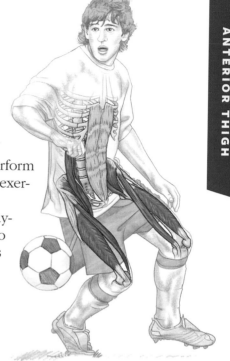

The hip flexor hold is also beneficial for soccer players. Although short passes do not commonly lead to hip flexor injuries, shots or long passes and crosses do. These latter types of kicks require the hip flexors to undergo a large stretch and immediately concentrically contract to kick the ball. By strengthening this muscle group, the muscles are better able to tolerate these types of kicks, making hip flexor injuries less common.

VARIATION

Cable Hip Flexion

Balancing on one foot, place the other foot in a strap attached to a cable resistance machine. Flex your hip until the top of the thigh is parallel to the floor; allow the thigh to return to the starting position by controlling the hip extension. Hip flexion with a cable involves the same motion as the hip flexor hold, but instead uses both concentric (during the upward movement) and eccentric (during the downward movement) muscle actions.

Note: One exercise that appears in chapter 8 requires special mention here: The leg extension is an excellent exercise to improve the strength of the quadriceps muscle group. Please refer to chapter 8 for instruction on how to perform this important exercise.

COPENHAGEN HOLD

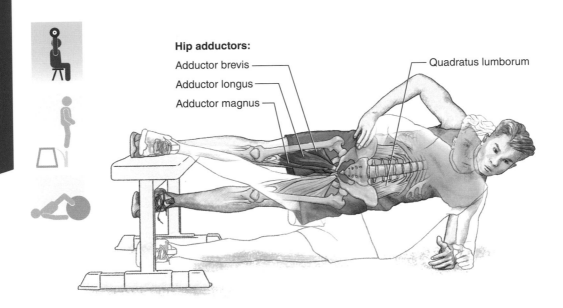

Hip adductors:

Adductor brevis

Adductor longus

Adductor magnus

Quadratus lumborum

Execution

1. Lie propped on your elbow on one side with the inside of the top ankle resting on a bench. Keep your opposite foot on the floor for support and balance.
2. Lift your hips in the air until there is a straight line from your top foot to your top shoulder.
3. Hold this position for a prescribed period.
4. Slowly lower to the starting position.
5. The illustration here is showing a Copenhagen hold progression of the Copenhagen hold with leg lift as described in the variation section.

Muscles Involved

Primary: Hip adductors (adductor longus, adductor magnus, adductor brevis) (top lower extremity)

Secondary: Quadratus lumborum (bottom lower extremity)

PREVENTIVE FOCUS

This is a difficult exercise requiring great strength of the hip adductor muscles. The combination of isometric hold at the top of the movement and the muscle force required to lift the hips and pelvis off the floor improve the strength and muscle endurance of the hip adductors of the top lower extremity.

The hip adductors are especially important for hockey players because they are responsible for helping to stabilize the hip joints when stopping. Up to 10 percent of hockey players injure their hip adductor muscles during the course of a season (Tyler et al. 2010). Although it is common to attribute these injuries to a lack of flexibility, the primary cause is more often related to hip adductor weakness. The hip abductor muscles are generally responsible for propulsion and are not commonly injured in hockey players.

VARIATION

Copenhagen Hold With Leg Lift

The original Copenhagen hold involves the use of the lower extremity to provide stability; because of this, it requires less muscle hip adductor muscle force to perform. One variation is to lift the hips as with the Copenhagen hold, but while maintaining that upper position, slowly lift the lower foot to the bench and back down for a prescribed number of repetitions. Each time the bottom foot is off the floor, the top hip adductor muscles must generate greater force to perform the exercise.

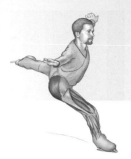

KNEE

The knee is one of the most studied, researched, and discussed joints in the body. Two possible reasons for this attention are the complex nature of the joint and its high rate of injury. The knee comprises three separate bones—tibia, femur, and patella—and two separate joints, the tibiofemoral and the patellofemoral, which are both covered in this chapter. Though many potential injuries to these joints may occur, special attention will be paid to the most frequently injured structures as well as the most common mechanisms for those injuries.

Note: All muscles acting at the knee joint are covered in other chapters (specifically the quadriceps and hamstrings in chapter 7). Although those muscles are referred to multiple times in this chapter, please refer to those chapters for detailed discussion of the muscles themselves and exercises for preventing injuries to those muscles.

TIBIOFEMORAL JOINT

The knee is commonly referred to as a *hinge joint*, and though other motions also occur—specifically internal and external rotation—its primary motions are flexion and extension. These motions occur at the tibiofemoral joint—the articulation between the tibia and femur—and are accomplished with activation of hamstrings (flexion) and quadriceps femoris (extension). Between these two bones, there are two types of cartilage: articular cartilage and the menisci. Articular cartilage covers the joint surface to provide smooth motion. The medial and lateral menisci are C-shaped, wedgelike pieces of cartilage that serve to deepen the tibiofemoral joint. This increased congruency helps support and protect the joint, guide motion, and provide some cushioning (see figure 8.1).

In addition to the stability provided by the menisci, the joint capsule surrounds the tibiofemoral joint and provides an additional degree of stability. Four primary ligaments also stabilize the tibiofemoral joint: anterior cruciate ligament (ACL), posterior cruciate ligament (PCL), lateral collateral ligament (LCL), and medial collateral ligament (MCL). The first three ligaments are distinct structures, whereas the last—MCL—is more muted in shape and structure. Each of these ligaments has a specific function.

129

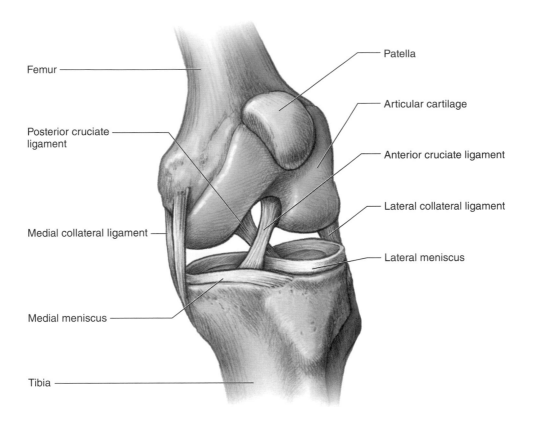

Femur

Patella

Articular cartilage

Posterior cruciate ligament

Anterior cruciate ligament

Lateral collateral ligament

Medial collateral ligament

Lateral meniscus

Medial meniscus

Tibia

FIGURE 8.1   Left knee ligaments and tissues.

- *ACL*. The ACL consists of two bundles, the anteromedial and posterolateral bundles, and travels from the posterior part of the medial aspect of the femur's lateral condyle anterior and lateral to the anterior tibial spine on the tibia, where it blends with the medial meniscus. It lies in front of (anterior) and crosses (cruciate) the PCL. ACL prevents anterior translation of the tibia on the femur (i.e., it prevents the tibia from moving forward in relation to the femur) and also prevents hyperextension. In addition to these motion restrictions, it also provides proprioceptive feedback to the nervous system.

- *PCL*. The PCL is posterior to the ACL and prevents posterior translation of the tibia on the femur and also prevents hyperextension. The PCL is not injured as often as the ACL.

- *MCL*. This ligament is located medially (toward the midline of the body) to connect the tibia and femur and prevents valgus (inward) movement of the knee in relation to the foot. Though this ligament is a common source of tibiofemoral injury, it is not as distinct as the other three tibiofemoral ligaments and does not often require surgery, unless it has been completely torn (grade III).

- *LCL*. Located laterally (away from the midline of the body), the LCL prevents varus (outward) knee motion. This ligament provides this support via its attachments to the fibula and the femur.

Because one of the most common tibiofemoral joint injuries involves the ACL, a lot of research has been performed to determine causes, best surgical techniques, evidence-based rehabilitation, and—more recently—prevention for this injury.

ACL Tear

An ACL tear is a devastating knee injury that commonly occurs when participating in sports requiring frequent high-impact landing and twisting, like soccer, basketball, football, and volleyball. Despite the amount of research performed and published over the past several years,

- the rate of ACL tears has not decreased,
- the number of athletes able to return to previous activity following ACL tear has not improved,
- the risk of post-traumatic osteoarthritis for those suffering an ACL tear is high,
- those who tear their ACL and have surgery are often unable to return to their previous activity level (Ardern et al. 2014),
- tearing the ACL puts athletes at an increased risk for unfavorable weight gain (Myer, Faigenbaum, et al. 2013; Whittaker 2015),
- athletes who tear their ACL report greater levels of disability (Cameron et al. 2013), and
- approximately 30 percent of athletes who tear their ACL have a related injury within the first two years (Paterno et al. 2014).

Given these dire statistics, it is incumbent both for providers and coaches to develop programs that reduce the risk of ACL injury and to maximize program participation and compliance by athletes. Recent research showed an overall 50 percent reduction in the risk of all ACL injuries and a 67 percent reduction for noncontact ACL injuries in females when participating in an injury prevention program (Webster and Hewett 2018). Unfortunately, these programs are underused, with fewer than one-third of youth soccer coaches having their athletes participate in an ACL injury prevention program (Finch et al. 2016; Mawson et al. 2018).

Several injury prevention programs have been developed, but no one program has been shown to be more effective than another (Huang et al. 2020). It is safe to say that doing some supplemental strength and conditioning of any kind is likely helpful. There is some evidence that an effective ACL injury prevention program should include the following:

• Increasing strength of the hamstrings and hip abductors (Grindstaff and Potach 2006; Khayambashi et al. 2016; Palmieri-Smith 2009; Zebis et al. 2009)

• Reducing inward motion of the knee (dynamic valgus) when landing, decelerating, jumping, and changing direction (Hewett et al. 2005; Myer et al. 2008, 2011; Paterno et al. 2010; Quatman and Hewett 2009)

• Increasing the amount of knee flexion upon landing (Myer et al. 2011)

• Improving overall strength, endurance, and fitness—though not universally accepted, this is likely a benefit (Collins et al. 2016; Dickin et al. 2015; Frank et al. 2014; O'Connor et al. 2015; Shultz et al. 2015; Sugimoto et al. 2015; Tamura et al. 2016)

PATELLOFEMORAL JOINT

The patellofemoral joint is the articulation between the floating patella—or kneecap—and the femur that lies behind it (see figure 8.2). The patella rests and functions within the trochlear groove of the femur. Though floating, the patella is held in place by both the walls of the trochlear groove and the patellar retinaculum, a collection of ligaments that provide stability. The medial portion that specifically limits lateral movement of the patella is the medial patellofemoral ligament (MPFL).

During typical function, the patella glides superiorly with quadriceps contraction and inferiorly when the quadriceps relax. During quadriceps contraction, the patella acts as a pulley between the proximal and distal attachments of those muscles. By acting as a pulley, the moment arm—the distance between the joint axis and the line of force acting on that joint—is lengthened, thereby increasing mechanical advantage to allow the quadriceps to concentrically pull on the tibial tuberosity and extend the knee. This type of motion occurs when walking up stairs or straightening the knee while seated. This structure also allows the quadriceps to act eccentrically to slow movement and absorb shock, as when squatting down, walking down stairs, or landing from a jump.

A special note on muscle function must be made here. Some believe that a specific portion of vastus medialis— the vastus medialis obliquus or VMO—can be activated to improve patellofemoral alignment, thereby reducing pain for some and improving stability for others. The medial-to-lateral alignment of this portion of the vastus medialis suggest the VMO could indeed improve patellofemoral alignment. While the belief behind this makes sense, it is not supported by research and has two fundamental obstacles:

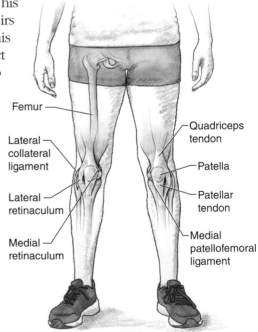

FIGURE 8.2 The patellofemoral joint comprises two bones, the patella and femur. The patella is held in place by a combination of muscle, other soft tissue restraints, and the shapes of both bones.

1. To date, research has not shown the VMO can be independently activated, regardless of how exercises are altered (e.g., change of foot or leg position) or what tools are used (e.g., ball between the knees, biofeedback).

2. There is limited, if any, evidence to suggest that this portion of vastus medialis has the ability to pull the patella medially to improve alignment.

Although many of the exercises used to reduce patellofemoral injuries are the same as those for the ACL, the types of injuries are unique. Some injuries occur because the patella does not move in the trochlear groove as designed, and some are due to repetitive use.

Patellar Instability

Patellofemoral instability occurs when an athlete's patella moves out of the trochlear groove, typically to the outside (laterally). Patellar instability can occur when the patella moves out of the trochlear groove and remains there until relocated—known as *dislocation*—or when the patella moves out of the trochlear groove but returns to the groove on its own—known as *subluxation* (see figure 8.3). There are several structures that help to keep the patella lying within the trochlear groove, including the shape of the groove, muscles, and ligaments—specifically the medial patellofemoral ligament (MPFL). The MPFL runs between the medial border of the patella and the medial epicondyle of the femur and is commonly torn in repeated episodes of instability, often requiring reconstruction.

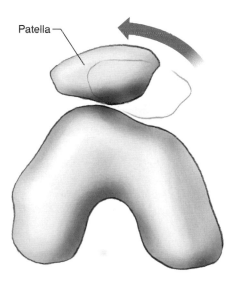

Patella

FIGURE 8.3 Lateral movement of the patella outside the trochlear groove. If the patella returns to the groove immediately, it is a subluxation. If the patella requires external repositioning, it is a dislocation.

Anterior Knee Pain

Anterior knee pain is often synonymously referred to as *patellofemoral pain syndrome*. But because more than the patellofemoral joint may be involved, *anterior knee pain* is a better general term to describe a variety of injuries. Some of these injuries include the following:

- Patellofemoral pain syndrome
- Chondromalacia patellae
- Osgood-Schlatter disease
- Sinding-Larsen-Johansson syndrome
- Synovial plica syndrome
- Patellar tendinopathy
- Pes anserine bursitis
- Quadriceps tendinopathy
- Prepatellar bursitis
- Iliotibial band syndrome

Anterior knee pain can occur for a variety of reasons and can be difficult to treat due to the variety of symptoms and locations involved. Risk factors for anterior knee pain include patella or femoral abnormalities, muscular weakness, and overuse. Generally, improving movement technique and strength of specific muscle groups (i.e., quadriceps and hip abductors) reduces the risk of anterior knee pain.

Patellar Tendinopathy

Patellar tendinopathy, commonly referred to as *jumper's knee*, is a specific type of anterior knee pain that (as the name suggests) involves the patellar tendon. This condition may or may not involve active inflammation; acute injuries to the patellar tendon do involve a release of inflammatory agents, but if the injury becomes more chronic or is a result of overuse, active inflammation is likely not present. Instead, chronic patellar tendinopathy more typically involves degenerative injury to the tendinous fibers, resulting in tendon pain and weakness. This pain is commonly felt when running (especially downhill), landing, and when descending stairs.

Because the risk factors for both knee joint–related injuries are similar, each of the ACL exercises in this chapter also reduce the risk of injury to the patellofemoral joint. Leg extension is included in this chapter specifically for patellofemoral joint injuries. It should be noted, however, that quadriceps weakness is a risk factor for subsequent injury following an initial ACL tear or surgery; therefore, the exercises listed for the patellofemoral joint in this chapter should be included in secondary ACL injury prevention programs as well.

Jumping and Landing Position

Many exercises in this chapter describe jumping and landing positions. The position we advocate to maximize performance of the drills is with knees bent and aligned with the second and third toes (see figure 8.4). It is acceptable (and natural) for the knees to move past the toes; however, this movement can be considered more advanced, so when beginning the squatting, jumping, and landing exercises described in this (and other) chapters, limit that forward motion to a position level with the toes. More advanced athletes can, and should, allow the knees to move past the toes.

Note: The knees should not move excessively inward (valgus movement) or outward (varus movement). Dynamic valgus is a known risk factor for knee injuries, including ACL tear.

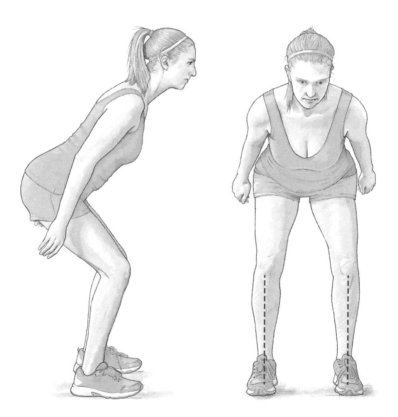

FIGURE 8.4 Proper plyometric landing position. *(a)* When viewed from the sides, the athlete's shoulders are in line with her knees, which helps to place the center of gravity over the body's base of support. *(b)* When viewed from the front, the athlete's knees are over her toes; excessive inward (valgus) movement increases the athlete's risk of lower extremity injury.

SINGLE-LEG SQUAT

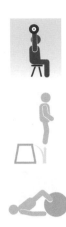

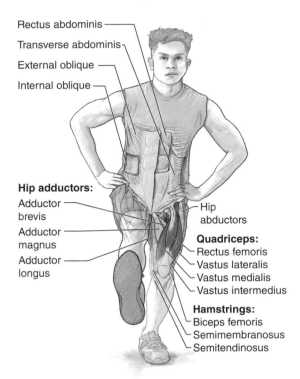

Rectus abdominis
Transverse abdominis
External oblique
Internal oblique

Hip adductors:
Adductor brevis
Adductor magnus
Adductor longus

Hip abductors

Quadriceps:
Rectus femoris
Vastus lateralis
Vastus medialis
Vastus intermedius

Hamstrings:
Biceps femoris
Semimembranosus
Semitendinosus

Execution

1. With your feet shoulder- to hip-width apart and your toes slightly pointed outward, lift your right foot off the floor.

2. Allow your left hip and knee to slowly flex while keeping the torso-to-floor angle constant.

3. *Note:* Maintain a flat-back position with your chest up and out. Keep your left heel on the floor and your knee aligned with the second and third toes of the foot.

4. Continue allowing your hips and knees to flex until your thigh is parallel to the floor or you are unable to lower any further.

5. Extend the hip and knee of the left foot, still keeping the torso-to-floor angle constant.

6. *Note:* Continue to maintain a flat-back position with your chest up and out. Keep your left heel on the floor and your knee aligned with the second and third toes of the foot.

7. Continue extending the hip and knee to reach the starting position.

Muscles Involved

Primary: Gluteus maximus, hamstrings (semitendinosus, semimembranosus, biceps femoris), quadriceps (rectus femoris, vastus lateralis, vastus medialis, vastus intermedius)

Secondary: Hip abductors, hip adductors (adductor longus, adductor magnus, adductor brevis), erector spinae (iliocostalis, longissimus, spinalis), rectus abdominis, external and internal obliques, transverse abdominis

PREVENTIVE FOCUS

The single-leg squat involves the use of all the thigh muscles and, to be performed correctly, requires proper lower body and trunk alignment. This maximizes the demands placed on the muscles involved. When performing, pay special attention to the knee performing the exercise; there is a tendency for that knee to "collapse" into a valgus position. This inward movement is termed dynamic valgus and is a risk factor for both tibiofemoral and patellofemoral injury. Performing this exercise as described reinforces the need for muscle recruitment during such tasks.

Any athlete in a sport that requires a partial squat position on a single lower extremity will benefit from the single-leg squat. Examples of this movement include planting the foot to drive off when changing direction in football, when kicking in soccer, and when responding to an offensive or defensive player in basketball. For athletes in these sports, incorporating a single-leg squat into their training programs will reinforce the proper positioning and alignment while also strengthening the muscles involved in those movements.

VARIATION

There are several variations of the single-leg squat (e.g., pistol squat, Bulgarian split squat, skater's squat) for the athlete to consider; one of those variations is provided here.

Levitating Lunge

The levitating lunge is performed the same way as the single-leg squat, but with the lifted knee positioned behind the other knee. From this position, the goal of the downward movement phase is to lower until the posterior knee just touches the floor (it should not rest on the floor and should not hit the floor forcefully).

STABILITY BALL HAMSTRING CURL

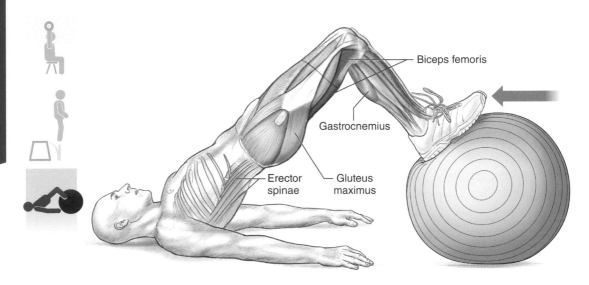

ANTERIOR CRUCIATE LIGAMENT

Biceps femoris

Gastrocnemius

Erector spinae

Gluteus maximus

Execution

1. Lying supine on the floor with feet on a ball.
2. Abduct your arms approximately 30 degrees.
3. Lift the hips off the floor to position so your feet, knees, hips, and shoulders are in a straight line.
4. Flex your knees to bring your heels toward your hips (this will cause the ball to roll backward).
5. Still keeping your hips and shoulders in a straight line, continue flexing your knees to a 90-degree angle; the soles of the feet will finish near the apex of the ball.
6. Allow your knees to extend and the ball to roll forward to the starting position.

Muscles Involved

Primary: Hamstrings (semitendinosus, semimembranosus, biceps femoris)

Secondary: Gluteus maximus, gastrocnemius, erector spinae (iliocostalis, longissimus, spinalis)

PREVENTIVE FOCUS

Proper hamstring function is important for sporting activity, but it also helps to protect and stabilize the tibiofemoral joint—as mentioned earlier, one of the ACL's functions is to prevent anterior translation of the tibia on the femur. Increasing strength of the hamstrings therefore reduces the risk of ACL injury (Myer et al. 2009). This exercise is unique because it involves both the proximal (hip) and distal (knee) portions of the hamstrings, though the focus is more on the distal knee motion as compared to the proximal action at the hip.

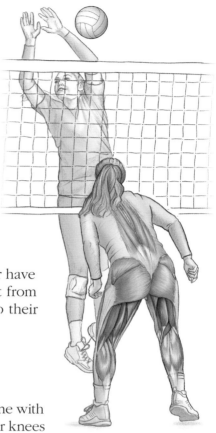

Athletes in sports that involve sprinting or who are at risk of ACL injury benefit from this type of hamstring exercise. Volleyball players in particular have a high incidence of ACL injury and would benefit from incorporating the stability ball hamstring curl into their programming.

VARIATION

Seated Leg Curl

This variation requires you to sit in a leg curl machine with your ankles resting on top of the roller pad and your knees lined up with the axis of the machine. Flex your knees as far as possible, then slowly allow them to extend back to the starting position. This exercise allows greater resistance to be used than the stability ball curl, which requires more trunk control to perform.

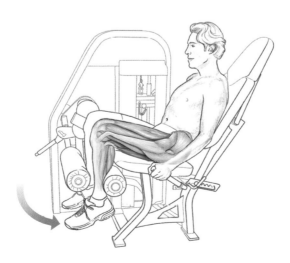

DECELERATION

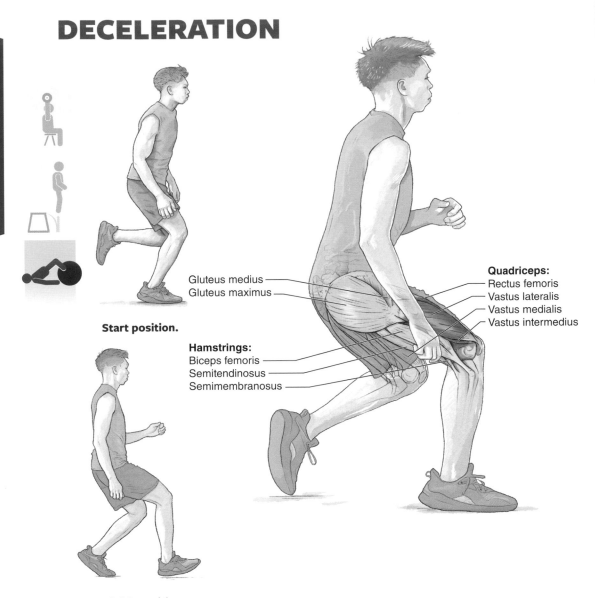

Start position.

Gluteus medius
Gluteus maximus

Quadriceps:
Rectus femoris
Vastus lateralis
Vastus medialis
Vastus intermedius

Hamstrings:
Biceps femoris
Semitendinosus
Semimembranosus

Finish position.

Execution

1. Run forward at half speed for approximately 20 meters.
2. Decelerate and stop within three steps, making sure to drop your hips low and keep your trunk upright.
3. As your ability to effectively control deceleration improves, increase to three-quarters speed and stop within five steps.
4. Finally, run at top speed and stop within seven steps.

Muscles Involved

Primary: Quadriceps (rectus femoris, vastus lateralis, vastus medialis, vastus intermedius)

Secondary: Hamstrings (semitendinosus, semimembranosus, biceps femoris), gluteus maximus, gluteus medius, gluteus minimus

PREVENTIVE FOCUS

Deceleration drills are intended to improve braking ability (specifically quadriceps function) and to assist in transfer of training from traditional strength exercises to more sport-specific movements. Training athletes to dissipate forces through practiced deceleration has repeatedly been shown to decrease the risk of ACL injury, whereas higher ground reaction forces, especially when experienced by those with less training age or experience (Bates et al. 2013), increases an athlete's risk of ACL injury during tasks requiring rapid stopping movement (Hewett et al. 2005; Miranda et al. 2013; Sell et al. 2007; Yu et al. 2006). Most sports and positions require deceleration from a sprint or with changes of direction, such as the following:

- A volleyball player running to the net
- A basketball player running to defend an inbound pass
- A soccer defender running to cut off a pass

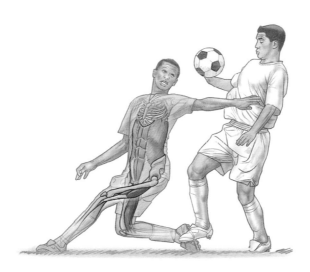

VARIATIONS

Two exercises which can be considered variations of the deceleration exercise—or exercises that improve the skill and physical requirements of deceleration—are the drop freeze and stability hop. Both of these exercises require you to slow and stop movement—i.e., decelerate—in a short amount of time.

(continued)

ANTERIOR CRUCIATE LIGAMENT

DECELERATION *(continued)*

Drop Freeze

Step from a box and absorb the landing by flexing your knees and landing as quietly as possible on both feet. Your knees should be lined up over your second and third toes, as shown in the landing position illustration in the sidebar on page 135.

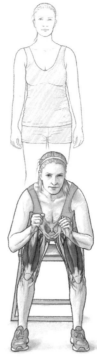

Stability Hop

Jump forward off one foot and land on the other foot, absorbing the landing by flexing your knee and landing as quietly as possible. Your knee should be lined up over your second and third toes. This is an excellent exercise to work on lower extremity alignment as well as to prepare for quick direction changes using proper technique.

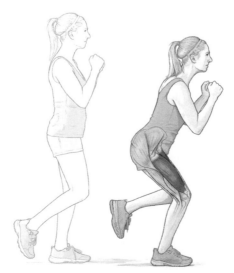

DROP (DEPTH) JUMP

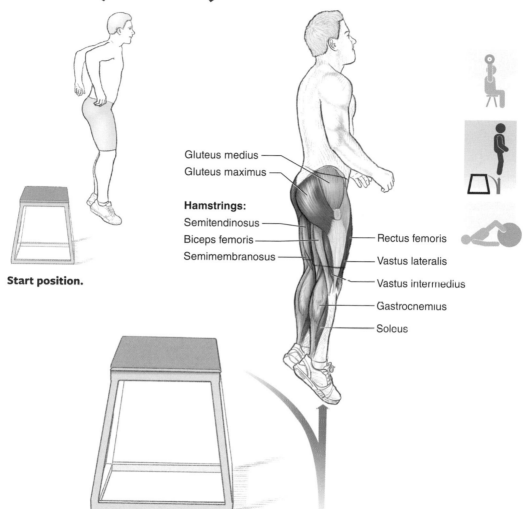

Start position.

Gluteus medius
Gluteus maximus

Hamstrings:
Semitendinosus
Biceps femoris
Semimembranosus

Rectus femoris
Vastus lateralis
Vastus intermedius
Gastrocnemius
Soleus

Execution

1. Assume a comfortable upright stance on a 12-inch (30 cm) box with your feet shoulder- to hip-width apart and your toes near the edge of the box.

2. Step from the box and land on the floor with both feet.

3. Upon landing, immediately jump up as high as possible, keeping your time on the ground as short as possible.

4. Land in the same position and absorb the landing by flexing your knees and landing as quietly as possible.

5. *Note:* Your knees should maintain proper alignment over the second and third toes of each foot.

(continued)

DROP (DEPTH) JUMP   *(continued)*

Muscles Involved

Primary: Quadriceps (rectus femoris, vastus lateralis, vastus medialis, vastus intermedius), gluteus maximus, soleus

Secondary: Hamstrings (semitendinosus, semimembranosus, biceps femoris), gluteus medius, gluteus minimus, gastrocnemius

PREVENTIVE FOCUS

Lower extremity plyometric exercises add speed and impact components not occurring in many other exercise modes. This particular exercise has two primary benefits: It reinforces proper knee alignment and it mimics the type of movement and impact experienced during sporting activities. By incorporating intense exercises into a training program, athletes are better conditioned to tolerate the demands of sport, including explosiveness and deceleration.

Most sports and positions require deceleration when landing from a jump, such as the following:

- A football wide receiver landing after catching a ball
- A basketball forward landing after grabbing a rebound
- A soccer defender landing from a header
- A volleyball blocker landing after a block at the net

VARIATIONS

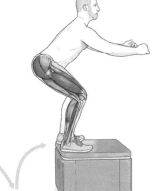

Drop (Depth) Jump to Second Box

This exercise is performed the same way as the drop (depth) jump; upon landing, however, the immediate jump up is onto a second box. The distance of the second box from the first will depend on your ability and experience with plyometric exercise; a distance of 24 inches (60 cm) is a good starting point (NSCA 2016).

Drop (Depth) Jump to 90-Degree Turn

This exercise is performed the same way as the drop (depth) jump; upon landing, however, immediately jump and turn your body 90 degrees as you land. As with the drop (depth) jump, you should absorb the landing by flexing the knees and landing as quietly as possible.

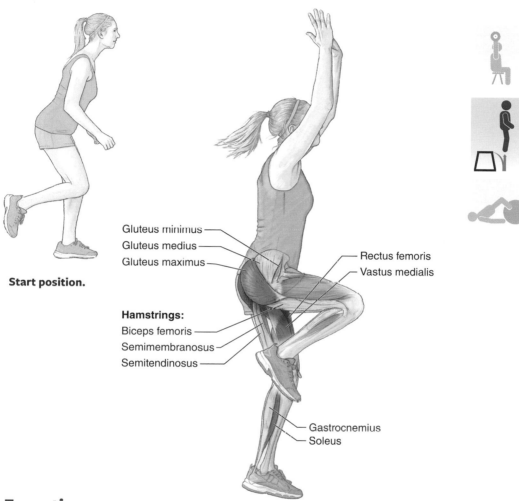

SINGLE-LEG VERTICAL JUMP

Start position.

Gluteus minimus
Gluteus medius
Gluteus maximus

Hamstrings:
Biceps femoris
Semimembranosus
Semitendinosus

Rectus femoris
Vastus medialis

Gastrocnemius
Soleus

Execution

1. Assume a comfortable, upright stance on one foot. Hold the free leg in a stationary position with the knee flexed throughout the exercise.

2. Squat down slightly, then immediately and explosively jump up, using both arms to assist and reach for a target.

3. Land on one foot in the starting position using proper knee alignment (see figure 8.4), and absorb the landing by flexing the knee and landing as quietly as possible.

4. Repeat the jump using the same leg.

5. *Note:* You should recover after each jump (i.e., repetitions are not continuous).

(continued)

SINGLE-LEG VERTICAL JUMP *(continued)*

Muscles Involved

Primary: Quadriceps (rectus femoris, vastus lateralis, vastus medialis, vastus intermedius), gluteus maximus, soleus

Secondary: Hamstrings (semitendinosus, semimembranosus, biceps femoris), gluteus medius, gluteus minimus, gastrocnemius

PREVENTIVE FOCUS

Like the drop (depth) jump, this plyometric exercise both focuses on proper knee alignment and mimics sport-specific movement and impact. By using only a single leg, however, this exercise requires the muscles in the jumping leg to produce more force, thus increasing the intensity as well as requiring greater balance and greater control of the jumping knee.

Dancers of all genres require periods of time functioning or landing on a single leg, such during leaps, jetes, and even turn variations. All dancers would benefit from using the single-leg vertical jump to improve alignment and strength while also reducing injury risk.

VARIATIONS

Single-Leg Vertical Jump—Continuous

The continuous variation of the single-leg vertical jump is performed the same way as the single-leg vertical jump, but the recovery period between jumps is minimized: Upon landing from one jump, immediately jump again without resting. This requires more control of the knee, and its continuous nature more closely mimics the activity occurring during most sports.

Single-Leg Side-to-Side Hop

Like the continuous variation of the single-leg vertical jump, the single-leg side-to-side hop is performed continuously, but instead of jumping vertically, the motion is to the side and then back to the starting position. To perform, place two markers 12 inches (30 cm) apart and stand on one. Using one leg, jump up and laterally to the other marker; upon landing, immediately jump to the starting marker again without resting. This requires more control of the knee, and its continuous nature more closely mimics the activity occurring during most sports.

SIDE HURDLE JUMP

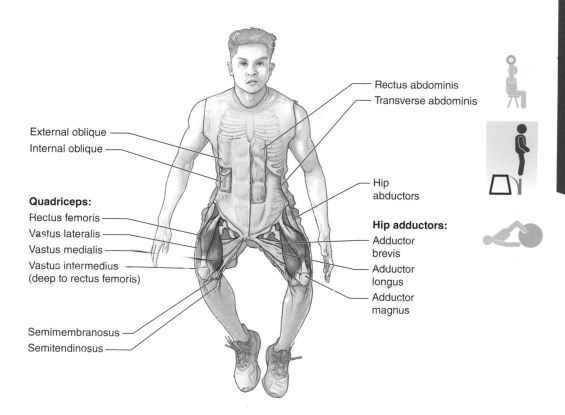

Rectus abdominis

Transverse abdominis

External oblique

Internal oblique

Hip abductors

Quadriceps:

Rectus femoris

Vastus lateralis

Vastus medialis

Vastus intermedius
(deep to rectus femoris)

Hip adductors:

Adductor brevis

Adductor longus

Adductor magnus

Semimembranosus

Semitendinosus

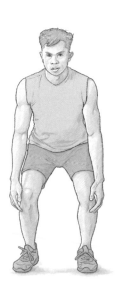

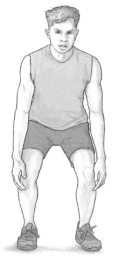

Start position.

Finish position.

(continued)

SIDE HURDLE JUMP   *(continued)*

Execution

1. Stand to the side of a hurdle with your feet shoulder- to hip-width apart.
2. While maintaining proper knee alignment (see figure 8.4), bend your knees slightly and jump up and over the hurdle with your legs together.
3. Land on both feet and absorb the landing by bending your knees and maintaining proper knee alignment.
4. Return to starting position and repeat.
5. *Note:* This may be performed by starting from either side of the hurdle.

Muscles Involved

Primary: Gluteus maximus, hamstrings (semitendinosus, semimembranosus, biceps femoris), quadriceps (rectus femoris, vastus lateralis, vastus medialis, vastus intermedius)

Secondary: Hip abductors, hip adductors (adductor longus, adductor magnus, adductor brevis), erector spinae (iliocostalis, longissimus, spinalis), rectus abdominis, external and internal obliques, transverse abdominis

PREVENTIVE FOCUS

The side hurdle jump—both the two-leg exercise and single-leg variation—adds a lateral component to jumping and requires the athlete to control both the jumping and landing positions in a way that differs from vertical jumps. This type of motion is common in several sports positions, but one of the most common is a football running back. These athletes often run straight ahead, then stop by landing on both feet and change direction by driving off one or both lower extremities. By performing the side hurdle jump with correct form and alignment, the athlete is better prepared for the cutting and changes of direction common in football.

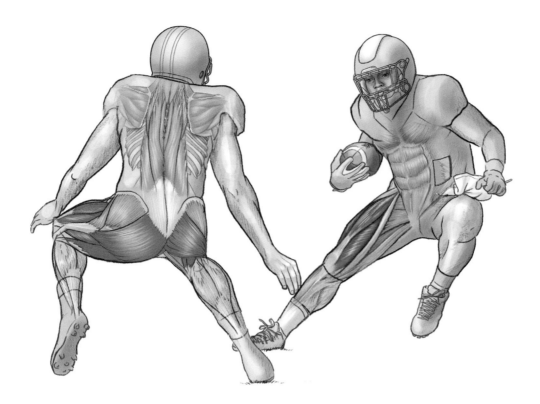

VARIATIONS

Side Hurdle Jump—Continuous

The side hurdle jump can be performed in a continuous manner as well: Upon landing from one jump, immediately jump over the hurdle again (in the opposite direction) without resting. This requires more control of the knees, and its continuous nature more closely mimics the activity occurring during most sports.

Single-Leg Side Hurdle Jump

Another common variation is to perform the side hurdle jump on a single leg. Standing next to the hurdle on one foot, jump up and over, landing on the same leg. This is a very challenging exercise and requires more control of the knee; because of the increased intensity, lowering the height of the hurdle is advised.

STANDING LONG JUMP TO SINGLE-LEG LANDING

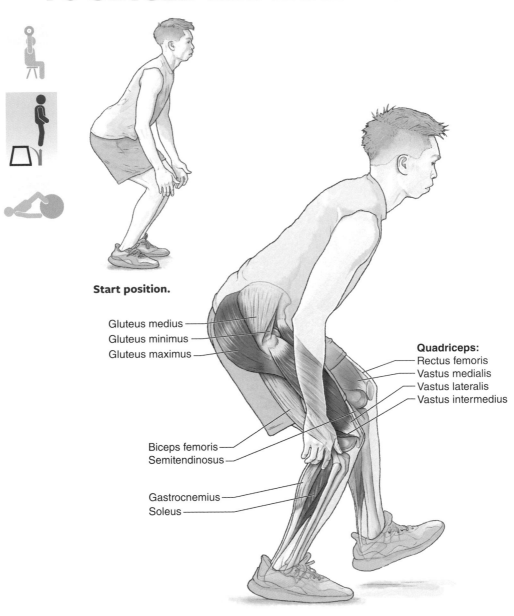

Start position.

Gluteus medius

Gluteus minimus

Gluteus maximus

Quadriceps:
Rectus femoris
Vastus medialis
Vastus lateralis
Vastus intermedius

Biceps femoris
Semitendinosus

Gastrocnemius
Soleus

Execution

1. Begin in a half-squat position with your feet shoulder- to hip-width apart.
2. Slightly squat down and immediately and explosively jump up and forward as far as possible with both feet, using your arms to assist with the jump.
3. Land on one foot in the starting position using proper knee alignment (see figure 8.4), and absorb the landing by flexing the knee and landing as quietly as possible.
4. *Note:* Allow complete rest between repetitions.

Muscles Involved

Primary: Quadriceps (rectus femoris, vastus lateralis, vastus medialis, vastus intermedius), gluteus maximus, soleus

Secondary: Hamstrings (semitendinosus, semimembranosus, biceps femoris), gluteus medius, gluteus minimus, gastrocnemius

PREVENTIVE FOCUS

The explosive nature of this jump is similar to that required in sport and sprinting, and the single-leg landing also mimics the deceleration common in sport. Further, this exercise emphasizes proper landing technique, including absorption and alignment; these two technique focus areas have been demonstrated to reduce injury risk (Hewett et al. 2005; Miranda et al. 2013; Sell et al. 2007; Yu et al. 2006). Figure skating is a sport that requires frequent single-leg landings. Although the landing surface differs from most sports, single-leg landing requirements are generally the same at the knee joint. Adding the standing long jump to single-leg landing into the training plan of figure skaters is important to reduce knee injury risk.

VARIATION

Standing Long Jump to Vertical Jump

This variation begins as the previous exercise does, but you land with both feet and then immediately perform a vertical jump, then again land with both feet, absorbing the impact and landing as quietly as possible.

LEG EXTENSION

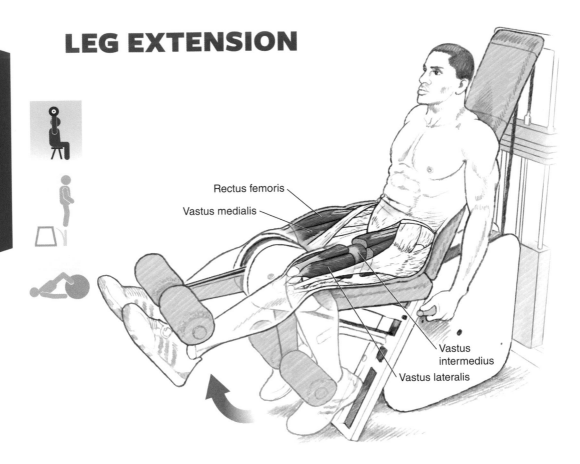

Rectus femoris

Vastus medialis

Vastus intermedius

Vastus lateralis

Execution

1. Sit on the machine with your knees aligned with the axis of the machine.
2. *Note*: If the back pad is adjustable, move it to align the knees with the axis of the machine and position the buttocks and thighs so that the backs of the knees are touching the front end of the seat.
3. Hook the front of the ankles under the ankle pad or pads.
4. *Note*: If the pad is adjustable, position it so it is in contact with the instep of the foot.
5. Keeping your thighs, lower legs, and feet parallel to each other, extend your knees until they are straight.
6. Allow your knees to slowly flex back to the starting position.

Muscles Involved

Primary: Quadriceps (rectus femoris, vastus lateralis, vastus medialis, vastus intermedius)

Secondary: None

PREVENTIVE FOCUS

This exercise has previously been viewed as controversial in the rehabilitation and injury prevention setting because of the notion that it is not "functional" and that it can cause a reconstructed ACL to loosen because of anterior shearing (which the ACL limits). However, it is the best exercise we are aware of to isolate the quadriceps. Because this motion is rarely used in sport or daily life, it can be viewed as nonfunctional; however, it is possible to perform more functional exercises (e.g., the back squat) but minimize use of the quadriceps muscles. This is especially important in building tolerance to loads at the patellar tendon and in reducing the risk of repeated ACL tears. Further, there is limited (if any) research that concludes any anterior shear that might occur has a deleterious effect to the ACL.

Any sport that involves the use of the lower extremities benefits from the inclusion of the leg extension exercise in a training program designed to reduce patellofemoral injury risk. Runners are a good example of athletes who commonly experience patellofemoral pain and would benefit from performing the leg extension. This is especially true when running downhill; there is a significant eccentric component involved in braking during downhill running.

VARIATIONS

Kettlebell Leg Extension

This exercise is very similar to the leg extension as described, but with two primary differences: It is a single-leg exercise, and it uses a kettlebell for resistance rather than a machine. For the kettlebell leg extension, sit with your thighs supported on a chair, bench, or box, and place the toes of one foot in the handle of a kettlebell. Maintaining contact with the sitting surface, extend your knee until it is straight, then allow your knee to slowly flex back to the starting position.

Nordic Quadriceps Exercise

Often referred to as the reverse Nordics, the Nordic quadriceps exercise is really the opposite of the hamstring variation—and, as its name indicates, its focus is on the quadriceps and not the hamstrings. To perform, begin in a tall kneeling position on the floor. Maintaining a straight line from your knees to shoulders, slowly lean back by flexing your knees. While lowering, you should start to feel a stretch in your anterior thighs. Continue leaning as far back as possible, then contract your quadriceps muscles to return to the starting position.

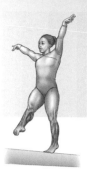

9

LEG, ANKLE, AND FOOT

The leg, ankle, and foot are three distinct anatomical areas with significant overlap and interaction among them (see figure 9.1). Each area and joint will be discussed, with specific muscle and joint considerations provided in each.

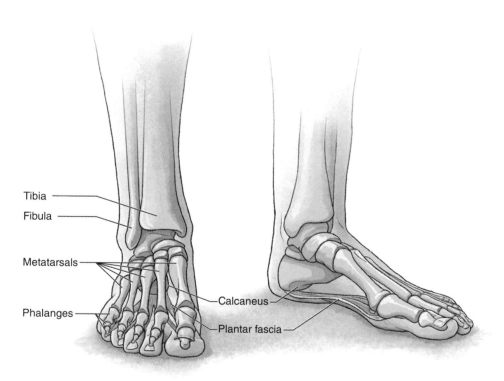

Tibia

Fibula

Metatarsals

Phalanges

Calcaneus

Plantar fascia

FIGURE 9.1 Anatomy of the leg, ankle, and foot.

LEG

The leg is the inferior part of the lower limb, between the knee and ankle joints. Although the entire lower limb is commonly referred to as the *leg*, only the area between the knee and ankle joints is the anatomical leg. The tibia and fibula are the bones of the leg, with the tibia being the primary weight-bearing bone of the leg. Superiorly, the tibia articulates—forms a joint with—with the condyles of the femur (covered in chapters 7 and 8) and inferiorly with the talus (covered later in this chapter). Though it does bear a small amount of weight, the main purpose of the fibula is to serve as a place of attachment for the muscles of the leg. The leg has three compartments—anterior, lateral, and posterior—with different muscles and structures in each.

The anterior compartment has four muscles, each of which is primarily concerned with dorsiflexion of the foot at the ankle joint and extension of the toes (see figure 9.2).

• *Tibialis anterior.* This muscle originates from the superior half of the lateral surface of the tibia and inserts at the base of the first metatarsal bone and medial cuneiform bone. Its primary function is dorsiflexion of the foot at the ankle joint, but it also inverts the foot. Though other muscles assist with these actions, tibialis anterior is the chief muscle to dorsiflex and invert the foot.

• *Extensor digitorum longus.* This muscle lies immediately lateral to tibialis anterior and forms four tendons, which diverge on the top of the foot to the lateral four toes. Originating from the lateral condyle of the tibia and superior three-quarters of the anterior surface of the fibula, extensor digitorum longus inserts on the middle and distal phalanges of the lateral four toes. As its name indicates, this muscle is responsible for extension of these toes. Because of its anterior location, it also assists with dorsiflexion of the foot at the ankle.

• *Peroneus tertius.* This muscle has its origin on the inferior third of the anterior surface of the fibula and inserts on the base of the fifth metatarsal bone (top side). Though it also assists with dorsiflexion, the primary function of peroneus tertius is eversion of the foot at the ankle.

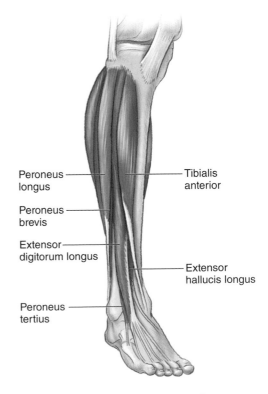

Peroneus longus

Peroneus brevis

Extensor digitorum longus

Peroneus tertius

Tibialis anterior

Extensor hallucis longus

FIGURE 9.2   Anterior muscles of the leg.

- *Extensor hallucis longus.* This muscle originates from the middle part of the anterior surface of the fibula and inserts on the base of the distal phalanx of the big toe. Its primary function is extension and hyperextension of the big toe, but it also assists with dorsiflexion of the foot.

The lateral compartment of the leg has only two muscles, both of which evert the foot. Both muscles lie posterior to the lateral malleolus; because of this position, both assist with plantarflexion (pointing the foot down) as well (see figure 9.2).

- *Peroneus brevis.* This muscle originates from the inferior 2/3 of the lateral surface of the fibula and inserts on the base of the fifth metatarsal bone and the tuberosity on the lateral side.

- *Peroneus longus.* This muscle originates from the head and superior two-thirds of the lateral surface of the fibula and inserts on the base of the first metatarsal bone and medial cuneiform bone (located behind the first meta-tarsal); these insertions are near those of tibialis anterior.

The posterior compartment of the leg has several muscles. The first three are more superficial and the second group of three are the deep muscles of the posterior leg compartment (see figure 9.3).

- *Gastrocnemius.* This is the most superficial muscle of the posterior compartment and has two heads: The lateral head originates from the lateral aspect of the lateral condyle of the femur and the medial head originates from the popliteal surface (area of the "back of the knee") of the femur, superior to the medial condyle of the femur. The two heads form a single muscle less than halfway down the calf, where it becomes a wide, flat tendon to insert on the posterior calcaneus via the Achilles tendon. The primary action of gastrocnemius is plantarflexion of the foot at the ankle joint. Because of its unique origin proximal to the knee, it also assists with flexion of the leg at the knee joint. However, any muscle that crosses two joints has a significant disadvantage when attempting to simultaneously act maximally at both joints, therefore, to plantarflex with maximal force, gastrocnemius must not be flexing the knee.

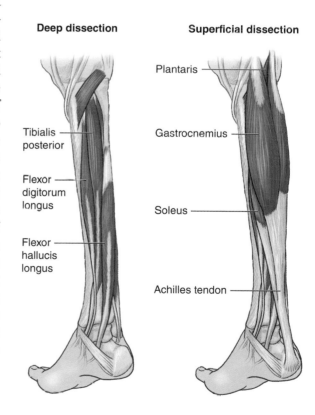

FIGURE 9.3   Posterior muscles of the leg.

- *Soleus.* Named for its resemblance to the sole fish, this muscle originates from the posterior aspect of the head of the fibula, superior 1/4 of the posterior surface of the fibula, soleal line of the tibia, and medial border of the tibia. Like gastrocnemius, it inserts on the posterior calcaneus via the Achilles tendon. As the largest muscle of the leg, soleus is a very strong muscle and works with gastrocnemius to plantarflex the foot at the ankle joint.

- *Plantaris.* This small muscle originates superior to the lateral condyle of the femur and the lateral head of the gastrocnemius and inserts on the posterior calcaneus, just superior to the insertion of the Achilles tendon. Though it can become injured, plantaris is primarily a proprioceptive organ and has minimal plantarflexion capabilities.

- *Flexor hallucis longus.* This deep muscle originates from the lower 2/3 of the posterior surface of the fibula and inserts on the base of the distal phalanx of the big toe and two sesamoid bones; these floating bones lie on either side of the tendon to protect it as it crosses the first metatarsal head. The flexor hallucis longus flexes the big toe and offers a limited amount of plantarflexion of the foot at the ankle joint.

- *Flexor digitorum longus.* This deep muscle originates from the posterior surface of the tibia, inferior to the origin of soleus, and inserts on the bases of the distal phalanges of the lateral four toes (i.e., toes 2-5). It flexes these toes.

- *Tibialis posterior.* This deep muscle originates from the posterior surfaces of both the fibula and tibia and inserts on the navicular tuberosity, cuneiform, and cuboid bones, and the bases of the second, third, and fourth metatarsal bones. Its primary action is supination and inversion of the foot (especially while plantarflexed) and offers a limited amount of plantarflexion of the foot at the ankle joint.

Because of their heavy use during both daily and sporting tasks, the most common injuries to the leg involve either muscles or tendons. These musculotendinous structures are used tens of thousands of times per day, and that number only increases with athletic practices or games.

Calf Strain

Strains to the gastrocnemius, soleus, and plantaris (collectively referred to as calf strains) occur in sports involving high-speed running, long distance running, and rapid acceleration and deceleration. Though injuries to the soleus are likely underreported (Draghi et al. 2021), strains in this area most commonly occur in either the medial head of the gastrocnemius or near the musculotendinous junction with the Achilles tendon. Gastrocnemius is a two-joint muscle like the hamstrings and rectus femoris muscles; because it functions at two joints and undergoes rapid changes, it may be more susceptible to injury. Athletes that are more likely to experience calf muscle strain include those participating in tennis, football, and running. On occasion, many will feel a pop in the posterior leg. This is sometimes referred to as *tennis leg* and, though it was originally thought to be an injury to plantaris (Powell 1883), it is more likely a strain of the medial head of gastrocnemius (Harwin and Richardson 2016).

Achilles Tendinopathy

The Achilles tendon is quite large and connects the gastrocnemius and soleus muscles to the calcaneus. Its size allows it to both resist great forces and to play an important role in transmitting force from those muscles to the foot and ankle. Irritation of this tendon is a common injury caused by repetitive energy storage and release. Though many refer to this as *Achilles tendinitis,* this term is misleading: As mentioned with the patellar tendon in chapter 8, the inflammation seen in injured tendons is unique and likely does not indicate a traditional inflammatory response. More than 50 percent of Achilles tendinopathies occur near the middle of the tendon, with a smaller portion—25 percent—occurring at its attachment to the calcaneus (De Jonge et al. 2011). More recent research has implicated plantaris as a contributor to reported Achilles pain (Olewnik et al. 2017). Activities that require repeated, forceful contractions of the calf muscles (e.g., running, basketball, soccer, football) are more likely to be associated with Achilles tendinopathy.

Shin Splints

Although calf muscle strains and Achilles tendinopathy occur posteriorly, pain on the anterior and medial aspects of the leg have been generally referred to as *shin splints*. Shin splints has been associated with each of the following structures:

- Tibialis anterior
- Tibialis posterior
- Flexor hallucis longus
- Flexor digitorum longus
- Tibial shaft
- Tibial periosteum

The medical diagnosis associated with shin splints is known as *medial tibial stress syndrome*. As such, the most commonly involved structures are tibialis posterior and the tibia. Tibialis posterior is responsible for slowing pronation (a combination of eversion, dorsiflexion, and abduction of the foot) when an athlete's foot contacts the ground; repeated landing without sufficient training of this muscle can lead to injury. When the tibia is involved, it can begin as an irritation of the periosteum and, if untreated, can progress to a stress fracture. It is most common in sports and activities involving running or repeated jumping and landing (e.g., dance) and is typically an overuse injury resulting from doing too much activity with too little training. There are several treatments for this diagnosis, but prevention—through thoughtful training and strengthening of specific muscles, like the tibialis posterior—is the preferred approach.

ANKLE

The ankle joint joins the leg and foot and is formed by three bones: the tibia and fibula of the leg and the talus of the foot. The tibia and fibula are connected by several ligaments and an interosseous membrane that runs between the two bones (see figure 9.4). Distally, they form a bracketlike socket known as a *mortise*. The talus of the foot articulates with the mortise formed by the tibia and fibula. The primary motions of the ankle are dorsiflexion and plantarflexion, but inversion and eversion also occur. It is these latter two motions that result in the majority of injuries at the ankle joint.

Laterally, the ankle derives stability from three separate ligaments: the anterior and posterior talofibular ligaments and the calcaneofibular ligament (see figure 9.4). These ligaments collectively resist and protect against inversion stresses. Medially, the ankle is stabilized by the stout deltoid ligament, which is comprised of four separate ligaments that form a triangle connecting the tibia to the foot (specifically the navicular, calcaneus, and talus bones). This group of medial ligaments resists and protects against eversion stresses.

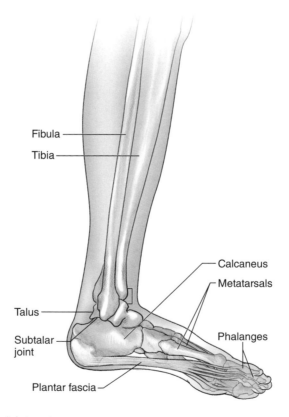

FIGURE 9.4   Ankle joint anatomy.

Though the ankle's structure of bones and ligaments would seem to provide sufficient protection against injury, this joint is one of the most commonly injured in sports. Because of this, extra attention is needed to reduce injury risk.

Ankle Sprain

Ankle sprains—a grade I, II, or III tearing of ligaments, depending on severity—are one of the most common injuries in sport (Fong et al. 2007) and can occur in three primary ways:

- *Inversion sprain.* This is the most common type of ankle sprain and occurs with extreme inversion; it is so common that it has been estimated that up to 70 percent of the general population have experienced an inversion ankle sprain during their lifetime (Hiller et al. 2012). This injury involves up to three lateral ligaments: anterior talofibular (the most frequently injured), calcaneofibular, and posterior talofibular. Inversion ankle sprains commonly occur in sports requiring quick, explosive changes of direction like basketball, soccer, volleyball, and football. A history of a previous inversion sprain is the greatest risk factor for this injury.

- *Eversion sprain.* Though the inside (medial) ankle ligaments—collectively the deltoid ligament—are strong, they can become injured with extreme eversion.

- *Syndesmotic sprain.* This is also referred to as a *high ankle sprain* and involves the distal tibiofibular syndesmosis—the fibrous joint between the tibia and fibula—and other ligaments between the distal tibia and fibula. Though a syndesmotic sprain can occur with any ankle motion, the most common are extreme external rotation or dorsiflexion of the talus. This injury is common in football, ice hockey, skiing, and wrestling (Nussbaum et al. 2001).

FOOT

The foot can be divided into several regions, but the most common divisions are the hindfoot, the midfoot, and the forefoot. The hindfoot is just distal to (beyond) the ankle joint and stops at the talonavicular and calcaneal-cuboid joints (often collectively referred to as the *transverse tarsal joint*). The bones of the hindfoot are the talus and the calcaneus. The midfoot begins at the transverse tarsal joint and ends where the metatarsals begin. This is commonly referred to as the *tarsometatarsal* (TMT) joint. There are several joints of the midfoot, but many offer only limited movement. The five bones of the midfoot are the navicular, the cuboid, and the medial, middle, and lateral cuneiforms. The forefoot has five metatarsals, two sesamoid bones, and 14 phalanges. The four lesser toes each have proximal, middle, and distal phalanges, which improve their ability to grip and help with balance. The big toe, however, has only a proximal and distal phalanx, which provides stiffness that—provided it is not too stiff—helps with propulsion when walking, running, and sprinting.

The bones of the foot form three arches: the medial longitudinal arch, lateral longitudinal arch, and transverse arch. The arches help to absorb the shock produced during landing, running, and walking. Further, because they are flexible, they allow the foot to accommodate or adjust to uneven terrain. These arches are supported passively by the bones themselves, but also by various ligaments and the plantar aponeurosis (commonly referred to as the *plantar fascia*—see figure 9.1). Active support and movement of the arches is provided by several small intrinsic muscles.

Pronation and Supination

Special mention must be made of two foot and ankle motions given a lot of attention in publications and by medical professionals: pronation and supination. Pronation is three coordinated movements of the calcaneus and foot—calcaneal eversion, forefoot abduction, and ankle dorsiflexion—in each plane of motion (frontal, transverse, and sagittal). Supination is essentially the opposite of pronation and also involves three movements in each plane of motion—calcaneal inversion, forefoot adduction, and ankle plantarflexion. Pronation and supination are normal motions and do not indicate injury or abnormal movement mechanics. The foot has two important functions when walking and performing sporting activity (including running, sprinting, jumping, and landing). The first is to adjust the foot to alterations in the ground surface while reducing the impact experienced by the rest of the body following ground contact. This is pronation; without this coordinated motion, athletes are at risk for other lower body injury. However, in addition to absorbing shock and adapting to the surface, the foot must also transmit force from the muscles of the lower leg to provide propulsion during push-off. For this, the foot must function as a rigid lever. This is supination; without this, the muscles of the foot and leg would lose efficiency and risk injury by absorbing loads instead of transferring them into the ground.

There are many small muscles located entirely in the foot. These muscles help move the toes and stabilize the foot. Because they originate and insert within the foot (i.e., not proximal to the ankle), these muscles are collectively referred to as *intrinsic foot muscles* (see figure 9.5). Two of these muscles are located on the top of the foot (extensor hallucis brevis and extensor digitorum brevis), and the remaining 10 muscles are located on the plantar aspect of the foot. These plantar muscles help to abduct, adduct, and flex the toes

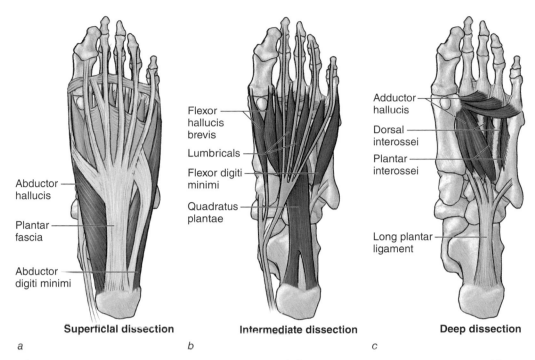

FIGURE 9.5 Intrinsic muscles of the foot: *(a)* superficial dissection; *(b)* intermediate dissection; *(c)* deep dissection.

and are (from superficial to deep): abductor hallucis, flexor digitorum brevis, abductor digiti minimi, quadratus plantae, lumbricals, flexor hallucis brevis, flexor digiti minimi, adductor hallucis, plantar interossei, and dorsal interossei.

Because of its inherent mobility and important role in daily life and sport, several injuries can occur in the foot. One of the most common involves the superficial connective tissue, the plantar fascia.

Plantar Fasciitis

Plantar fasciitis is painful irritation of the plantar fascia at its origin on the medial calcaneal tuberosity. Though traumatic injury is possible, this is more commonly an overuse injury and tends to occur in athletes who perform large volumes of running, like long distance runners and soccer players. Foot posture—specifically overpronation—has been linked with plantar fasciitis. However, the research on this is mixed, with some studies finding an association (Aranda and Munuera 2014) and other studies concluding there is not a relationship (Landorf et al. 2021).

HEEL RAISE

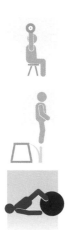

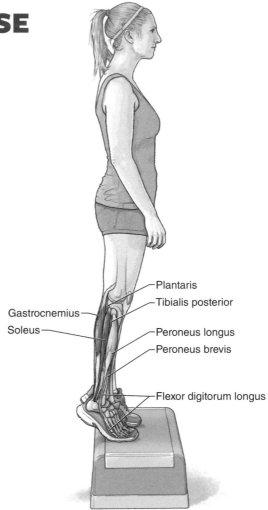

Plantaris

Tibialis posterior

Gastrocnemius

Soleus

Peroneus longus

Peroneus brevis

Flexor digitorum longus

Execution

1. With the balls of your feet positioned at the edge of a step, stand with your feet and legs parallel to each other and your knees straight.

2. Allow your heels to drop down lower than the step in a comfortable, stretched position.

3. Keeping your knees straight and feet parallel, fully plantarflex your feet and ankles to rise up on your toes.

4. Allow your heels to slowly lower back to the starting position.

5. *Note:* Avoid rolling your ankles outward at the top of the motion.

Muscles Involved

Primary: Gastrocnemius, soleus

Secondary: Plantaris, tibialis posterior, flexor digitorum longus, flexor hallucis longus, peroneus longus, peroneus brevis

PREVENTIVE FOCUS

The ankle plantarflexors are involved in countless sporting activities, including the explosive actions of jumping, sprinting, and changing direction. as well as acting eccentrically when decelerating and absorbing the forces when landing. By targeting these muscles, the plantarflexors (specifically gastrocnemius and soleus) and Achilles tendon are better conditioned to tolerate the aforementioned stressors.

Gymnastics requires its athletes to rise up onto their toes during several activities. Leaping during a tumbling pass, sprinting on the vault, turns on the balance beam, and dismounting from all apparatuses involve the muscles involved in the heel raise. Whether the goal is control, propulsion, or even eccentric function (as during a landing), performing the heel raise helps strengthen the posterior leg muscles and tendons, prepare other structures of the foot and ankle to tolerate those types of movements, and reduce the risk of foot and ankle injury.

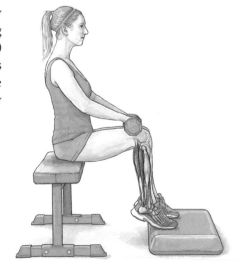

VARIATIONS

Single-Leg Heel Raise

This exercise is performed the same way as the heel raise, but with only one leg at a time. By using only one lower extremity, the single-leg heel raise is more intense and challenging than the standard heel raise.

Seated Heel Raise

The seated heel raise is performed the same way as the heel raise, but in a seated position. Sit on a chair (or in a special seated heel raise machine) with your thighs parallel to each other, knees flexed to 90 degrees, and the balls of your feet at the edge of a step. You may place a weight on the top of each thigh for additional resistance. Allow your heels to drop down lower than the step in a comfortable, stretched position; fully plantarflex your feet and ankles, and then allow your heels to slowly lower back to the starting position. By sitting with your knees flexed to 90 degrees, this limits the ability of the gastrocnemius to perform the exercise and allows the soleus to be the primary muscle involved, which is especially important for running-focused activities.

POGO

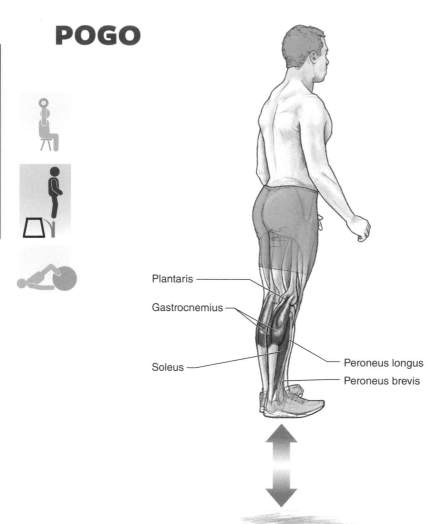

Plantaris

Gastrocnemius

Soleus

Peroneus longus

Peroneus brevis

Execution

1. Assume a comfortable, upright stance with your feet shoulder- to hip-width apart.

2. Using your arms and shoulders to assist with the motion, jump up using only the lower portion of your legs. This involves slight flexion and extension of the knee but relies primarily upon plantarflexion of the ankle and foot.

3. Once in the air, dorsiflex your ankles.

4. Land on your full feet, then immediately jump back up, with most of the motion coming from the ankle and foot joints.

5. *Note:* To maximize movement elasticity, maintain the described locked position of the feet throughout to ensure sturdy contacts and quick, elastic takeoffs. Minimize horizontal and lateral movements (forward and backward or side-to-side).

Muscles Involved

Primary: Gastrocnemius, soleus

Secondary: Plantaris, tibialis posterior, flexor digitorum longus, flexor hallucis longus, peroneus longus, peroneus brevis, quadriceps (rectus femoris, vastus lateralis, vastus medialis, vastus intermedius)

PREVENTIVE FOCUS

There are several benefits to the pogo exercise. One of the primary purposes is to enhance landing and takeoff mechanics from the ankle, as well as the knee and hip. In addition, this exercise helps you to direct forces downward into the ground; this impact (and resultant ground reaction force) is an important stressor the body must learn to navigate.

The pogo helps prepare the muscles and tendons for sprinting by preferentially targeting the ankle and foot with repeated hops instead of the knee and hip. Further, having the athlete dorsiflex the ankles during the flight phase of this exercise helps reinforce the efficient "toes up" position during sprinting.

VARIATION

Single-Leg Pogo

This exercise is performed the same way as the pogo, but on a single leg. Assuming the same comfortable, upright stance, flex one thigh at the hip with the ankle dorsiflexed. Your knee should be held above hip level, with your heel in front of the supporting knee. Using your arms and shoulders in an upward motion, jump up using only the lower portion of the standing leg. Land on the full foot, then immediately jump back up, with most of the motion coming from the ankle and foot joints.

SKIP

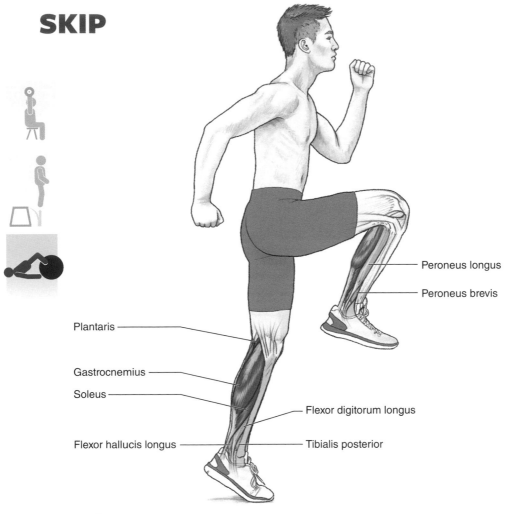

Peroneus longus

Peroneus brevis

Plantaris

Gastrocnemius

Soleus

Flexor digitorum longus

Flexor hallucis longus

Tibialis posterior

Execution

1. Lift one leg to approximately 90 degrees of hip and knee flexion.
2. Begin with a countermovement on one leg and jump up and forward on that leg. The free leg should remain in the starting flexed position until landing.
3. Land in the starting position on the same leg.
4. Immediately repeat the skip with the opposite leg.

Muscles Involved

Primary: Gastrocnemius, soleus

Secondary: Plantaris, tibialis posterior, flexor digitorum longus, flexor hallucis longus, peroneus longus, peroneus brevis

PREVENTIVE FOCUS

The skip is a very good exercise to work on the muscles that help you stride while also helping to direct forces downward into the ground; this impact (and resultant ground reaction force) is an important stressor the body must learn to navigate. One other benefit is to train the muscles, joints, and other structures to tolerate the quick impacts and rebounds required in many sports and reinforce the explosiveness required when sprinting and performing other sporting motions. Every athlete in sport that involves running benefits from the skip.

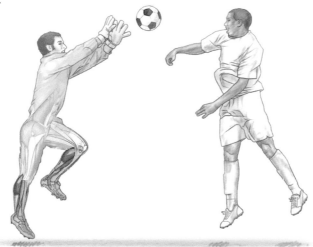

VARIATIONS

There are several variations for the skip, but three are the fast skip, backward skip, and side skip.

Fast Skip

The fast skip, though similar to the traditional skip, is more closely related to a drill to improve acceleration mechanics. The focus here is to emphasize the upward drive of the knee of the free leg during the swing and the hip extension from the stance leg. As you drive the lead toes up, the bottom of your foot should graze the ground as it swings forward. The movement finishes with the foot under the posterior thigh. The focus of the fast skip is extension of the thigh, recovery, high cadence, and forward propulsion (not distance).

Backward Skip

This exercise is performed the same way as the skip, but the initial (and subsequent) jump is backward instead of forward. By jumping backward, there is an added degree of coordination required. Further, there is a greater eccentric load on the Achilles tendon and involved muscles during each landing.

Side Skip

This exercise is performed the same way as the skip, but the initial (and subsequent) jump is lateral instead of forward. This exercise also requires greater coordination and also challenges the ankle joint of the lead leg to tolerate inversion stress without injury.

RELEVÉ HOLD

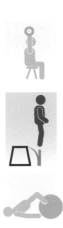

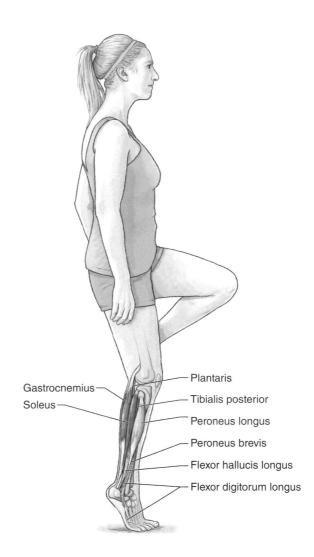

Gastrocnemius

Soleus

Plantaris

Tibialis posterior

Peroneus longus

Peroneus brevis

Flexor hallucis longus

Flexor digitorum longus

Execution

1. With your feet and legs parallel to each other, lift one leg to approximately 90 degrees of hip and knee flexion.

2. Keeping the stance knee straight, fully plantarflex that foot and ankle to rise up on your toes.

3. Maintain this position for the prescribed time, then allow the heel to slowly lower back to the starting position.

4. *Note:* Avoid rolling the ankles outward at the top of the motion.

Muscles Involved

Primary: Gastrocnemius, soleus

Secondary: Plantaris, tibialis posterior, flexor digitorum longus, flexor hallucis longus, peroneus longus, peroneus brevis

PREVENTIVE FOCUS

Relevé is a dance term that means "to rise up." Though traditionally performed with the feet turned out and starting in a bent knee position (i.e., plié), we use the term *relevé hold* to describe a heel raise that is held at the top. Performing isometric exercises helps to strengthen and improve the muscular endurance of the plantarflexors (specifically gastrocnemius and soleus) and the Achilles tendon, which is a necessary component of many activities.

Ballet dancers are very prone to foot and ankle injuries. Sometimes this is due to poor technique (e.g., sickling, or rolling the ankle outward, during relevé); sometimes it is simply the repetitive nature of ballet. Performing the relevé with proper form as part of a training program is one way to reduce that risk of injury. Adding a hold at the top of the movement both reinforces the proper position and, via the associated isometric contraction, helps to strengthen the muscles, tendons, and other structures involved. Though the movement is specific to ballet and even gymnastics, the relevé hold should be included in all Achilles tendon or ankle injury prevention programs.

VARIATION

Relevé Landing Hold

In this variation, you jump up with both feet and land on one foot in the relevé position. Upon landing, maintain this position for a specified period of time. Like the relevé hold, this variation improves muscular endurance, but the landing introduces impact, a stressor athletes frequently encounter in sport.

RESISTANCE BAND INVERSION

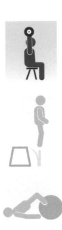

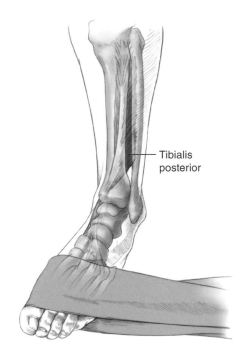

Tibialis posterior

Execution

1. Sit on a table, bench, or floor with your legs straight in front of you.
2. Loop a resistance band around the inside of one foot; the other end can be affixed to a post or held by a partner.
3. Keeping the resistance band around the inside of your foot and without allowing your leg or thigh to move, slowly move the foot inward as far as is comfortable.
4. Slowly allow the foot to move outward as far as is comfortable.

Muscles Involved

Primary: Tibialis posterior

Secondary: Tibialis anterior

PREVENTIVE FOCUS

Tibialis posterior is an important muscle because it helps to invert the ankle, but more importantly, it acts eccentrically to slow pronation of the foot when landing from a jump or when running. This muscle, like tibialis anterior, has been associated with shin splints. Runners would benefit from this inversion exercise.

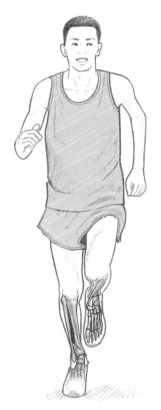

VARIATION

Resistance Band Inversion With Plantarflexion

This exercise is performed the same way as resistance band inversion, but with the ankle plantarflexed throughout the motion. This position better isolates tibialis posterior, because tibialis anterior is unable to offer the same assistance.

HEEL WALK

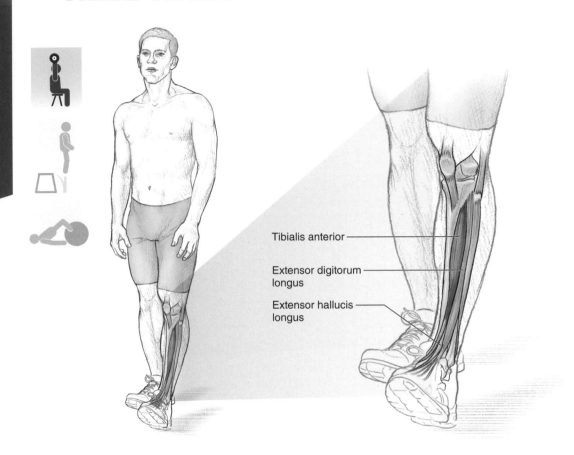

Tibialis anterior

Extensor digitorum longus

Extensor hallucis longus

Execution

1. Assume a comfortable, upright stance with your feet shoulder- to hip-width apart.
2. Dorsiflex your ankles to lift the toes and balls of both feet off the ground.
3. Maintaining this foot and ankle position, walk a specified distance.

Muscles Involved

Primary: Tibialis anterior

Secondary: Extensor digitorum longus, extensor hallucis longus

PREVENTIVE FOCUS

By strengthening the ankle dorsiflexors, athletes are able to prepare these muscles for sporting activity. Specifically, these muscles dorsiflex (lift) the ankle during the flight phase of running and sprinting and help to control and slow ankle plantarflexion with each contact with the ground while running. As with resistance band inversion, running is an obvious sport whose athletes would benefit from practicing the heel walk in training programs. By strengthening the anterior muscles, they are better able to tolerate the repeated dorsiflexion required when running.

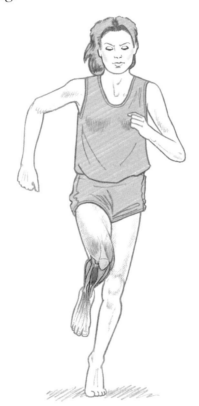

VARIATION

Manual Eccentric Dorsiflexion

Sit on a table, bench, or floor with your leg in front of you, knee straight. Have a partner grasp the top of the foot and pull it down into a plantarflexed position while you resist this motion. This exercise results in a strong eccentric muscle action of the ankle dorsiflexor. As mentioned previously, this is important to help control ankle plantarflexion just after initial contact with the ground when running. Therefore, this can be used as a sport-specific exercise.

RESISTANCE BAND EVERSION

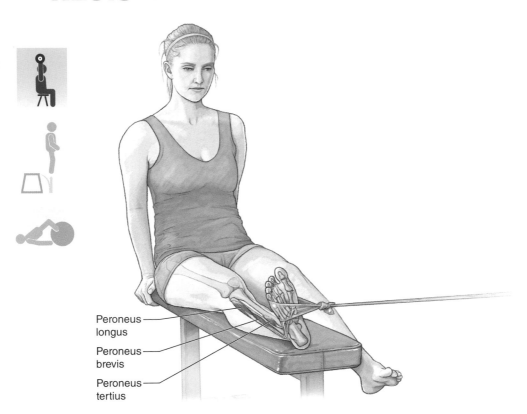

Peroneus longus

Peroneus brevis

Peroneus tertius

Execution

1. Sit on a table, bench, or floor with your leg straight in front of you.
2. Loop a resistance band around the outside of the foot; the other end can be affixed to a post or held by a partner.
3. Keeping the resistance band around the outside of your foot and without allowing your leg or thigh to move, slowly move the foot outward as far as is comfortable.
4. Slowly allow the foot to move inward as far as is comfortable.

Muscles Involved

Primary: Peroneus longus, peroneus brevis, peroneus tertius
Secondary: None

PREVENTIVE FOCUS

Inversion ankle sprains are very common in sports that require frequent changes of direction or running on uneven terrain. For example, trail runners often encounter either holes or obstacles such as exposed roots or rocks. When encountering these, the ankle may invert farther than the joint structure allows, resulting in a sprain of the lateral ankle ligaments. Strengthening the ankle evertors improves overall ankle stability, which is especially helpful in reducing the risk of an inversion ankle sprain.

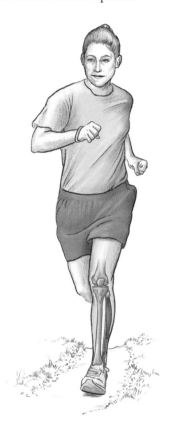

VARIATION

Isometric Eversion

Assume the same seated position with your feet straight out in front of you and place the outside of your foot against an immovable object, like a wall. Without allowing your leg and thigh to move, push the outside of your foot into the wall with as much effort as possible. Hold for a specified period, relax, and repeat. Like resistance band eversion, this exercise works on the strength of the ankle evertors. By using an isometric muscle action, the potential to generate greater force is possible.

SHORT FOOT

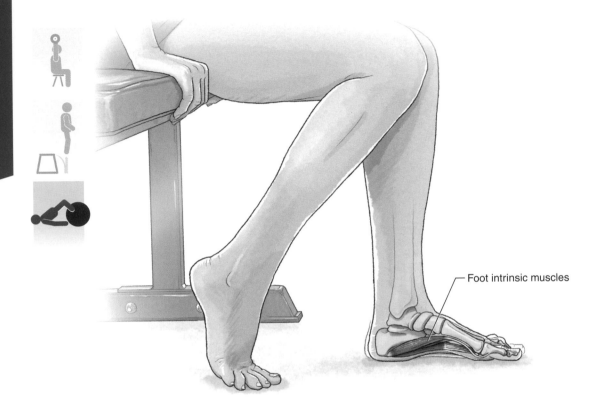

Foot intrinsic muscles

Execution

1. Sit with your knees flexed to 90 degrees and your ankle in a neutral position.
2. Without curling your toes, attempt to bring the head of the first metatarsal (the bone in the foot just behind the big toe) toward the heel (i.e., "shorten" the foot).
3. *Note*: The forefoot and heel should not get off the ground.

Muscles Involved

Primary: Foot intrinsic muscles (extensor hallucis brevis, extensor digitorum brevis, abductor hallucis, flexor digitorum brevis, abductor digiti minimi, quadratus plantae, lumbricals, flexor hallucis brevis, adductor hallucis, flexor digiti minimi, plantar interossei, dorsal interossei)

Secondary: None

PREVENTIVE FOCUS

Training the intrinsic foot muscles has been demonstrated to reduce the risk of running-related injuries by more than two times (Taddei et al. 2020). Performing these exercises will help to reduce the risk of injury to all athletes who perform a lot of running, sprinting, jumping, and landing.

The short foot exercise (and the following variation) help to strengthen the intrinsic foot muscles. By doing this, those muscles are better able to support all of the foot's arches and joints, thereby reducing the risk of foot injuries. Because ballet dancers experience frequent foot injuries, they would particularly benefit from this exercise.

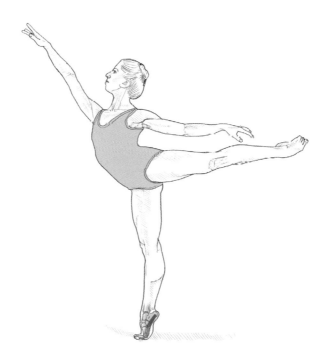

VARIATION

Arch Lift

Though similar to the short foot exercise, the arch lift focuses on increasing the arch height. In a seated position with your foot flat on the floor, raise the plantar arch in an arch shape. Keep your heel and toes on the ground.

BAREFOOT WALK

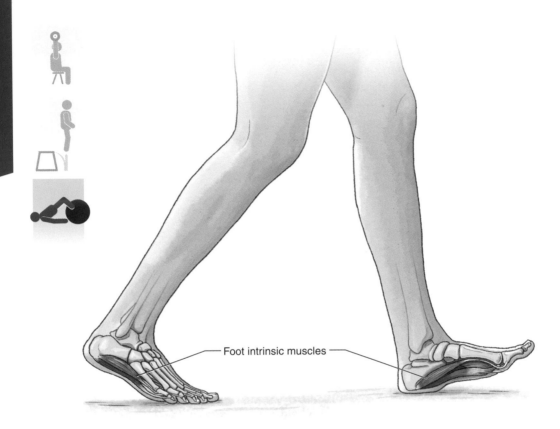

Foot intrinsic muscles

Execution

1. Remove your shoes and assume a comfortable, upright stance with your feet shoulder- to hip-width apart.
2. Begin walking forward at a comfortable, self-selected pace.
3. Continue for a specified distance or time; we suggest beginning with 5 minutes.
4. *Note:* Inspect the walking surface and area prior to removing shoes to be sure all debris and any dangerous objects are out of the walking path.

Muscles Involved

Walking uses many muscles. Those listed below are responsible for walking. When used to reduce foot and ankle injuries, it is those that are *italicized* this exercise focuses on.

Primary: Quadriceps femoris, hamstrings, gluteus maximus, gluteus medius, *gastrocnemius, soleus, flexor hallucis longus, flexor digitorum longus, tibialis posterior, tibialis anterior, extensor hallucis longus, extensor digitorum longus, peroneus tertius, peroneus brevis, peroneus longus, foot intrinsic muscles*

Secondary: Pectineus, adductor longus, adductor brevis, adductor magnus

PREVENTIVE FOCUS

Footwear can support the medial longitudinal arch and other structures of the foot. By removing footwear, the intrinsic foot muscles (and some extrinsic muscles, like tibialis posterior) must provide that support. In addition to runners, ballet dancers benefit from barefoot walking because it strengthens the intrinsic foot muscles and other muscles that help support the arch (i.e., tibialis posterior). It also helps to strengthen the other connective tissues and joint structures within the foot.

Note: Barefoot running has been discussed in the research literature and can be an efficacious training mode to challenge joint stability and improve running and muscular efficiency. However, the time required to begin such a program is beyond the scope of this textbook and will not be covered.

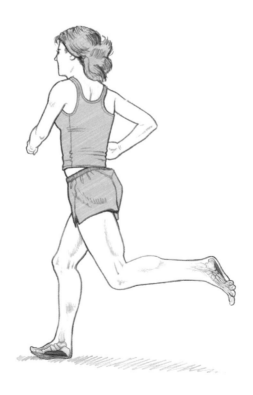

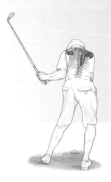

WARM-UP FOR INJURY PREVENTION

Warming up prior to physical activity is the standard method of preparing the body for exercise, training, or competition. Performing a warm-up can improve exercise and sport performance (Fradkin et al. 2010) and may reduce injury risk (Fradkin et al. 2006; McGowan et al. 2015; Shrier 1999, 2000; Silva et al. 2018). Some of the specific benefits include

- improved rate of force development (Asmussen et al. 1976; Swanson 2006),
- faster muscle contraction (Hoffman 2002),
- increased strength and power (Bergh and Ekblom 1979; Enoka 2015; Takeuchi et al. 2021),
- increased flexibility (Takeuchi et al. 2021),
- faster running speed (Gil et al. 2020),
- increased blood flow and oxygen delivery to involved muscles (McArdle et al. 2014), and
- enhanced mental preparedness (Bishop 2003).

However, it is important to determine the goals of the warm-up. Common goals include preparing for activity, improving flexibility, and reducing injury risk. This chapter will discuss the warm-up both as a way to prepare for movement as well as reduce injury risk. We will use a stepwise approach to take you from a general warm-up to an injury prevention warm-up to an activity-specific warm-up (Darrall-Jones et al. 2021; see figure 10.1). Each of these phases increases in intensity while also becoming more sport specific.

183

Stepwise Approach to Warm-Up

General Warm-Up

These exercises prepare athletes for activity by increasing the temperature of the general body through the use of common, general movements. Each of these exercises are performed at submaximal levels for 5 to 10 minutes.

Examples

1. Running
2. Cycling
3. Walking

Injury Prevention Warm-Up

The following exercises target commonly injured areas for specific sports. Exercises for the injury prevention warm-up are performed in 1 to 2 sets of 10 repetitions each.

Examples

1. Nordic hamstring curl (see chapter 7, page 117)
2. Side plank (see chapter 5, page 74)
3. Single-leg squat (see chapter 7, page 136)
4. Heel raise (see chapter 9, page 164)
5. Copenhagen hold with leg lift (see chapter 7, page 127)

Activity-Specific Warm-Up

These exercises provide activity-specific movements to prepare the athlete for practices and competition. The volume and intensity of these exercise varies, but for those listed here, 3 to 5 repetitions of 30 meters each is common.

Examples

1. Sprint
2. Skip (see chapter 6, p. 168)
3. Shuffle (see this chapter, p. 192)

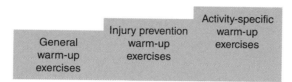

FIGURE 10.1 Warm-up order should progress from general to injury prevention to activity-specific warm-up exercises.

One last benefit of the warm-up—in particular the specific warm-up—is post-activation potentiation (PAP), a phenomenon by which force produced by a muscle is increased due to a previous contraction. In other words, provided the initial muscle contraction does not result in fatigue, brief muscle contractions involving high loads may increase muscle performance (Stone et al. 2008). A common example is performing a back squat, resting briefly, then jumping or sprinting. In this example, the back squat potentiates (or increases) the subsequent performance (the jump or sprint). This text will not cover PAP as part of the warm-up because the focus is on injury prevention, but this is a valuable technique to improve athletic performance.

GENERAL WARM-UP

A common general warm-up involves 5 to 10 minutes of activity designed to increase the athlete's heart rate to increase blood flow and oxygen to the involved muscles, as well as increase respiratory rates and improve joint fluidity (deVries and Housh 1995). This should be viewed as preparation for the injury prevention and activity-specific warm-ups to come. As the name indicates, the general warm-up typically includes activities that are general in nature, meaning they are not specific to a particular sport, exercise, or activity. However, the general warm-up likely looks different for different types of athletes. For example, athletes in a team sport like soccer or basketball might perform an easy five-minute run, whereas a weightlifter might ride a stationary bike for this time.

INJURY PREVENTION WARM-UP

Following the general warm-up, the injury prevention warm-up targets commonly injured areas with exercises designed to reduce the risk of those given injuries. These exercises are similar to those provided in chapters 3 through 9 in this text but are performed at non-fatiguing levels. Like the general warm-up, the injury prevention warm-up will differ based on the athlete's activity or sport. For example, a soccer player will include exercises to reduce ACL, hamstring, and ankle injuries, whereas a baseball player will perform exercises to reduce shoulder and elbow injuries.

Injury Prevention Warm-Up Programs

Several warm-up programs have been developed to target common causes of injuries. Examples of these programs include warm-ups for running, soccer, basketball, and gymnastics.

In addition to sport-specific injury prevention warm-ups, specific mention should be made of popular injury prevention warm-up programs focused on reducing the risk of ACL injuries. Two of the most often used ACL injury prevention programs include The Santa Monica Sports Medicine Research Foundation's PEP Program as well as 11+ (formerly known as FIFA 11+). Although different, these programs have similar approaches: Both require approximately 20 minutes to complete; both include running, strength, and plyometric exercises; and both have been shown to be effective at reducing injuries in the groups who adhere to the programs.

PEP

The PEP (Prevent injury and Enhance Performance) program was one of the first ACL injury prevention warm-up programs and "consists of a warm-up, stretching, strengthening, plyometrics, and sport specific agilities to address potential deficits in the strength and coordination of the stabilizing muscles around the knee joint" (Silvers and Mandelbaum 2001, p. 206). This program originally focused on female soccer players, but the movements and exercises are applicable to many other sports—like basketball, volleyball, and American football—as well (Herman et al. 2012; Noyes and Barber Westin 2012; Pollard et al. 2017; Rodríguez et al. 2018).

11+ (formerly known as FIFA 11+)

11+ has become one of the most popular ACL injury prevention programs used. Like the PEP program, 11+ has a soccer focus as it has been endorsed by the international governing body of soccer, Fédération Internationale de Football Association (FIFA), and its research section, FIFA Medical Assessment and Research Centre (F-MARC). However, the combination of running, strength, plyometric, and balance exercises incorporated in 11+ make it a nice program to reduce ACL injury risk and is recommended to be performed prior to all training sessions and games (Al Attar et al. 2016; Barengo et al. 2014; Herman et al. 2012; Mayo et al. 2014; Rössler et al. 2019; Silvers-Granelli et al. 2015).

ACTIVITY-SPECIFIC WARM-UP

Following the general and injury prevention warm-ups is the last warm-up phase before the scheduled activity begins—the activity-specific warm-up. This warm-up shifts to those movements that are common to the athlete's sport or activity and may include rehearsal of certain movements (Young and Behm 2002). It is performed at progressively increasing intensities and serves to prepare the specific muscles and movements required to achieve optimum neuromuscular performance (McArdle et al. 2014). Specific warm-up periods differ depending on the sport or activity. There are many approaches to specific warm-up periods; some examples include the following:

- *Sprinting:* Technique drills and specific movements (e.g., A-skip, single exchange, triple exchange), followed by slow to fast sprints of shorter distance
- *Tennis:* Upper and lower body exercises; bilateral and unilateral jumps; 10-second acceleration, deceleration, and change-of-direction drills (2-3 sets of 6-10 repetitions; approximately 5 minutes) (Fernandez-Fernandez et al. 2020)
- *Team field sports (e.g., soccer, handball):* Three 2-minute bouts of small-sided games with a passive recovery of 1 minute between bouts (Dello Iacono et al. 2021)

FLEXIBILITY AND THE WARM-UP

A common recommendation is to include flexibility exercises in the warm-up session. As discussed in chapter 2, flexibility is a combination of a joint's range of motion and the extensibility of the tissues surrounding the given joint. The most direct method to increase an athlete's flexibility is through stretching. There are three types of stretching:

1. *Static:* Passive movement held for a set amount of time, typically 10 to 30 seconds
2. *Dynamic:* Controlled movement into and out of a stretched position without holding at the end range
3. *Ballistic:* Combination of static and dynamic stretching in which an end position is reached, but movement (typically a bouncing movement) occurs

As mentioned in chapter 2, stretching—primarily static, but also dynamic—has been shown to acutely decrease power production for the short time after it has been performed (Gremion, 2005; Opplert and Babault, 2018; Sá et al. 2015; Yamaguchi et al. 2006; Young and Behm 2002). To our knowledge, there is no research to determine if stretching over a period of weeks or after activity results in the same loss of power production.

If athletes do not have sufficient range of motion or tissue extensibility to perform their given sport or activity at the time of warm-up, stretching to achieve that flexibility is warranted. Examples of athletes who require great flexibility include gymnasts, ballet dancers, and baseball pitchers. Athletes who have similar flexibility requirements would benefit from pre-activity stretching. If the athlete already possesses the necessary flexibility to perform the movements required, stretching is not required because there is little research to support the use of static or dynamic stretching to prevent injuries (Shrier 1999; Witvrouw et al. 2004).

Although stretching is not necessary for most athletes, we acknowledge that there is a tradition of stretching and that participating in group stretching activities might provide a team building opportunity for athletes. Therefore, we recommend that, when desired, stretching be performed after activity so as not to detrimentally affect strength and power production during practices and games.

WALKING LUNGE

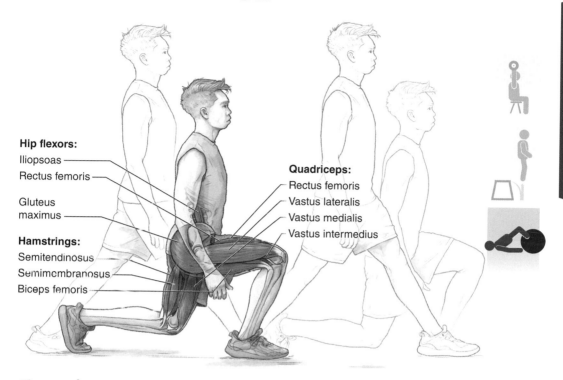

Hip flexors:
Iliopsoas
Rectus femoris

Gluteus
maximus

Hamstrings:
Semitendinosus
Semimembranosus
Biceps femoris

Quadriceps:
Rectus femoris
Vastus lateralis
Vastus medialis
Vastus intermedius

Execution

1. Planting your left foot flat, take an exaggerated step forward with your right foot.

2. Lower toward the ground by allowing your right hip and knee to slowly flex and your left foot to roll up onto the ball of the foot.

3. *Note*: As described in chapter 8, your right knee should be lined up with the second and third toes of your right foot—i.e., not too far inward, not too far outward—and may move beyond (forward of) your right foot. Your weight should be balanced evenly between the balls of your left and right feet, and your torso should remain upright and perpendicular to the ground.

4. Forcefully push up and forward by extending your right hip and knee.

5. Lift your left foot and immediately take an exaggerated step forward, repeating the steps above.

Muscles Involved

Primary: Gluteus maximus, hamstrings (semitendinosus, semimembranosus, biceps femoris), iliopsoas, quadriceps (rectus femoris, vastus lateralis, vastus medialis, vastus intermedius)

Secondary: None

INVERTED HAMSTRING STRETCH

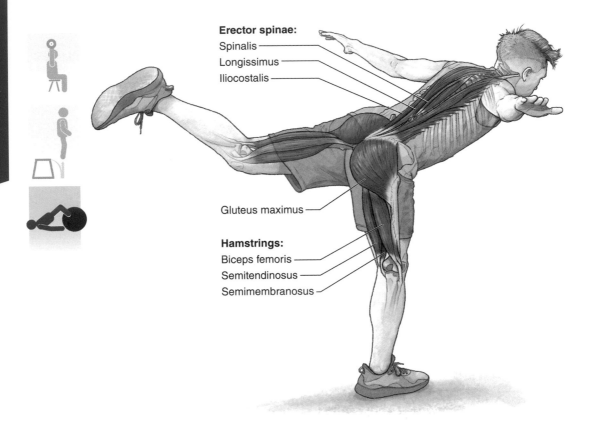

Erector spinae:
Spinalis
Longissimus
Iliocostalis

Gluteus maximus

Hamstrings:
Biceps femoris
Semitendinosus
Semimembranosus

Execution

1. Holding your arms out to the sides (90 degrees of shoulder abduction), bend forward at the waist while reaching and stepping back with the left leg.

2. *Note:* Avoid leaning to the side (i.e., pelvis should remain level). Your upper body should be almost parallel with the ground and you should feel a stretch in the right hamstrings.

3. Place your left foot on the ground and allow your upper body to return to an upright position.

4. Immediately repeat on the opposite side.

Muscles Involved

Primary: Hamstrings (semitendinosus, semimembranosus, biceps femoris), gluteus maximus, erector spinae (iliocostalis, longissimus, spinalis)

Secondary: None

SINGLE-LEG STAIR BOUND

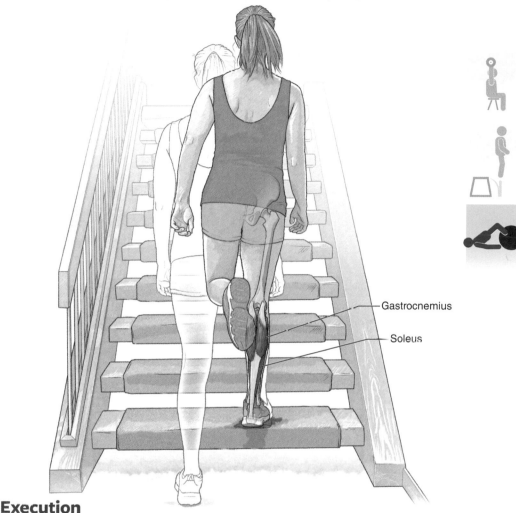

Gastrocnemius

Soleus

Execution

1. While standing on a set of stairs, drop backward to a lower step or the floor with your left foot.
2. As soon as your left foot contacts the lower step, immediately explode up and forward.
3. Land on the next step up with the right foot.
4. Repeat this sequence for the given distance or number of steps.
5. *Note:* As described in figure 8.4 on page 135, when landing, your knee should be lined up with the second and third toes of your foot—i.e., not too far in, not too far out.

Muscles Involved

Primary: Gastrocnemius, soleus, quadriceps (rectus femoris, vastus lateralis, vastus medialis, vastus intermedius), gluteus maximus

Secondary: None

SHUFFLE

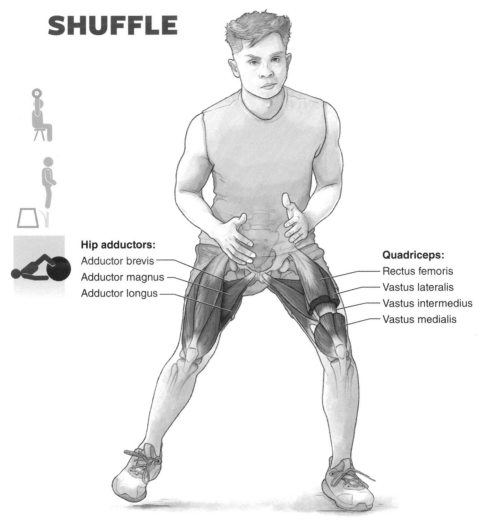

Hip adductors:
Adductor brevis
Adductor magnus
Adductor longus

Quadriceps:
Rectus femoris
Vastus lateralis
Vastus intermedius
Vastus medialis

Execution

1. Stand with your feet slightly wider than hip-width apart and your hips low with both knees flexed.
2. Using your right foot to push off, shuffle to the left.
3. Without allowing your feet to cross or touch, land on your left foot, then right foot, and immediately push off to the left with the right foot again.
4. Repeat for a prescribed distance.
5. *Note:* This movement should be similar to a glide, not a jump or hop.

Muscles Involved

Primary: Hip adductors (adductor longus, adductor magnus, adductor brevis), hip abductors, quadriceps (rectus femoris, vastus lateralis, vastus medialis, vastus intermedius)

Secondary: None

ANKLE FLIP

Execution

1. Jump forward off your right leg, leading with your left leg.
2. Land on your left foot and quickly rebound and jump forward, minimizing ground contact time and maximizing force projected into the surface.
3. *Note:* In addition to minimizing ground contact time, the focus of this exercise is to minimize knee flexion while keeping your ankle dorsiflexed. This exercise is really a running- or bounding-type motion that emphasizes the rebound off the surface by focusing on lower body—primarily ankle—elasticity.

Muscles Involved

Primary: Gastrocnemius, soleus

Secondary: None

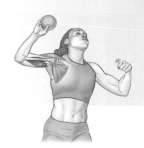

INJURY PREVENTION PROGRAM DESIGN

Effective injury prevention programs are similar to training programs designed to improve traditional measures of athletic performance, such as strength, power, and aerobic endurance. Just like traditional training programs, injury prevention programs require the manipulation of key variables that allow the body to adapt to the challenges presented to it, to improve the given outcome measure, and ultimately to reduce the risk of injury.

INJURY PREVENTION FOCUS STEPS

When designing a program to reduce the risk of injury, the focus is slightly different than that of a traditional training program. Both program design approaches start with the needs analysis, exercise selection, training frequency, training load and repetitions—i.e., intensity—and volume. When designing a program to reduce injury risk, ideal exercise order and rest periods between exercises have not been determined. These two variables are therefore not included. But a new variable—timing of the program—is listed. Therefore, the focus for injury prevention program design includes the following five steps:

1. Needs analysis
2. Exercise selection
3. Training frequency
4. Timing
5. Intensity and volume

In addition, it is important to be mindful of the three training principles: specificity, overload, and progression. First, as mentioned in chapter 2, the training must be specific to the movements common in the athlete's sport. In this case, the program design should also be specific to the structure or body region to which the athlete is trying to prevent injury and also consider the athlete's history of injury. Next, the program must challenge the athlete by providing sufficient stimulus (e.g., overload via increased weight or faster speed) necessary for adaptation. Lastly, the program must gradually and appropriately become more challenging through the deliberate management—i.e., progression—of select training variables.

The remainder of this chapter will briefly review the five focus steps that must be properly attended to in order to most effectively reduce the risk of injury. Each step will be discussed and put into context with examples of a step-by-step design of an ACL injury prevention program.

Step 1: Needs Analysis

When designing a program to reduce injury risk, it is important to evaluate the athlete's injury prevention needs. To do this, we conduct a needs analysis, which includes the following (see table 11.1):

- *Sport and anatomy evaluation.* Each sport and position has unique biomechanical or physiological requirements, and thus unique injury risks. Likewise, each anatomical structure is designed in such a way that unique movement, stabilization, and functional requirements exist. The goal of sport and anatomy evaluation is to determine these requirements (e.g., strength, muscle attachments and contraction types, speed of contraction, deceleration, changes of direction, joint structure).

- *Injury history.* Previous injury is one of the largest risk factors for both reinjury and subsequent injury. Reinjury is an injury following a previous injury to the same structure—for example, if an athlete sprains an ankle and then sprains the same ankle again three months later. Subsequent injury is any other injury that occurred after the initial injury—for example, if an athlete sprains an ankle and then injures the other (contralateral) ankle or an adjacent structure. Understanding an athlete's injury history can guide programming to address common reinjuries and subsequent injuries.

- *Goals and background.* Each athlete has a unique background and goals for both general and injury prevention training. This component of the needs analysis allows some flexibility when designing the injury prevention program.

TABLE 11.1 ACL Injury Prevention Program: Needs Analysis

SPORT AND ANATOMY EVALUATION	INJURY HISTORY	GOALS AND BACKGROUND
ACL runs from the femur to the tibia and resists anterior shear of the tibia in relation to the femur. **ALIGNMENT RISK FACTORS** Landing from a jump with a shallower knee flexion angle and greater dynamic valgus increases the risk of ACL injury. **BIOMECHANICAL RISK FACTORS** Increased knee joint loading increases the risk of ACL injury (Hewett et al. 2005; Myer et al. 2008, 2011; Paterno et al. 2010; Quatman and Hewett 2009). **STRENGTH** Weakness of the hamstrings and hip abductor muscles increase the risk of ACL injury (Ford et al. 2008; Khayambashi et al. 2016; Knapik et al. 1991; Myer et al. 2004, 2008; Söderman et al. 2001; Withrow et al. 2008). If previous injury has occurred, quadriceps weakness has been associated for increased risk of ACL injury and osteoarthritis.	Previous ACL injury increases the risk of both reinjury to the same ACL and subsequent injury to other structures within the same knee or to the contralateral ACL.	The goal of the program is to improve lower extremity alignment, specifically maximizing knee flexion and minimizing dynamic valgus upon landing and when decelerating and changing direction. In addition, improving the strength of the hamstrings and hip abductors reduces injury risk for those who have not had a previous ACL injury; improving quadriceps strength is important for those with previous ACL injury.

Step 2: Exercise Selection

In this step, we determine which mode of exercise will be chosen. As discussed in chapter 2, *exercise mode* refers to the type of exercise. The modes of exercise covered in chapter 2 are strength training, plyometric training, speed and agility training, flexibility training, and aerobic endurance training. The latter three will be grouped here under the heading of "special training exercises," which may be exercises specific to the sport or injury. Our training programs will focus on these modes of exercise. There is no specific research on the number of exercise modes to be included in an injury prevention program. In general, we recommend four to six strengthening exercises, three to four plyometric exercises, and up to four special training exercises, though this will vary based on the season (see table 11.2).

TABLE 11.2 ACL Injury Prevention Program: Exercise Selection

STRENGTH TRAINING EXERCISES	PLYOMETRIC TRAINING EXERCISES	SPECIAL TRAINING EXERCISES
Back squat	Drop (depth) jump	Running
Single-leg squat (and variations)	Drop (depth) jump to second box	Deceleration
Forward lunge	Standing long jump to single-leg landing	
Side lunge	Single-leg vertical jump	
Nordic hamstring curl		
Romanian deadlift		
Side plank		

Step 3: Training Frequency

Training frequency is the number of injury prevention sessions performed each week. Training frequency for general sports performance often changes depending on the time of the sporting year or season; the same is true with injury prevention training as well. Each season—preseason, in-season, and off-season—has a specific goal and training frequency (see table 11.3). The goal of the preseason is to maximize performance prior to competition and to prepare for the season ahead. General preseason preparatory conditioning has two important benefits: It reduces overall injury risk and improves performance (Myer et al. 2005, 2007; Myer, Ford, Brent, et al. 2006; Myer, Ford, McLean, et al. 2006).

Though they can be convenient, in-season injury prevention strategies can be limited. This phase tends to be performed at a lower intensity and is often considered a time to simply retain the improvements of technique gained during the preseason.

Because strength, power, and tolerance to stressors are important for injury prevention, off-season is the ideal time to develop a strong conditioning base for the more intense training that occurs during the preseason and in-season. Unfortunately, injury prevention strategies often end once the season ends. To be sure, it can be difficult from a scheduling standpoint to coordinate injury prevention sessions during this period, but we advocate for continuing to focus on technique while simultaneously training to improve muscular strength, power, and endurance. Each season of the sporting year is important, but programs that incorporate injury prevention programming into multiple seasons have the greatest positive impact on biomechanics and injury reduction (Gilchrist et al. 2008; Klugman et al. 2011; Myer GD, Stroube BW, DiCesare CA, et al. 2013; Stroube et al. 2013).

TABLE 11.3   ACL Injury Prevention Program: Training Frequency

SPORT SEASON	SESSIONS PER WEEK
Preseason	3
In-season	2
Off-season	4

Step 4: Timing

Injury prevention program timing is the placement or scheduling of injury prevention exercises when training. Injury prevention may be scheduled before practices, before games, after practices, or as standalone sessions. Timing decisions are most often based on convenience and how the injury prevention exercises affect the quality of games or other training sessions; they should be scheduled to allow for adequate recovery so that athletes do not become too fatigued to efficiently participate in upcoming practices or competitions. Several scheduling approaches are possible, but they can be best categorized as being performed with another training session (e.g., activity preparation or warm-up) or as a standalone training session (see table 11.4).

Most approaches to injury prevention training combine those exercises with other training sessions. When used, it is very common for injury prevention exercises to be performed prior to practice or games. Scheduling in this way is convenient and has been shown to increase compliance (Sugimoto et al. 2012). This is the method we advocate and outline how to do this in chapter 10. Performing exercises right after other training sessions is another option to consider (Potach et al. 2018). Not only is this convenient as well, there might be another added benefit: Decelerating, landing, and changing direction when fatigued may be an important component of injury prevention programs. Although this should not be done with all sessions, performing injury prevention exercises that focus on good alignment after other training sessions may provide additional novel stimulus.

Scheduling injury prevention exercise sessions as standalone training sessions, especially during the off-season, is a good option as well. Arranging the program in this way may allow athletes to better address strength, power, and tolerance to impact at intensities that are more likely to result in the sought-after adaptations to stressors (Augustsson 2013). The most important considerations, however, are compliance (Dix et al. 2020; Sugimoto et al. 2012) and allowing athletes to get the correct mode and quantity of exercise targeted to reduce injury risk (Sugimoto et al. 2012, 2015; Sugimoto, Myer, Barber-Foss et al. 2014; Sugimoto, Myer, Bush et al. 2014).

TABLE 11.4   ACL Injury Prevention Program: Timing

SPORT SEASON	SCHEDULE
Preseason and in-season	Before practice sessions as part of the warm-up
Off-season	Standalone sessions

Step 5: Intensity and Volume

Intensity is the relative difficulty of a given exercise or group of exercises and is most often measured by load (the amount of resistance used) or complexity. This is one of the most critical aspects of injury prevention program design. To achieve the desired adaptation, the program must provide both overload and progression. The intensity must be progressed to avoid plateaus in strength and motor control development (Augustsson 2013). With sufficient training load (>80% 1RM), most individuals can increase strength and power in less than six weeks (Goodwill et al. 2012; Oliveira et al. 2013; Weier et al. 2012).

Another way to increase training intensity is by varying exercise complexity and novelty. Early in the injury prevention training process, progressing the relative complexity of exercise may be enough to provide an appropriate challenge that leads to the desired gains. Focusing on exercise difficulty requires more movement exploration as compared to actual strength and power gains. Because technique and alignment are risk factors for many injuries, it is important to attend to these factors.

Exercise volume is the amount of work an athlete does during each session and may be measured in a variety of ways. Calculation of volume can include load, but for this text, we consider volume to be related only to the total number of repetitions performed during an injury prevention session (see table 11.5; Fleck and Kraemer 2014; McBride et al. 2009; O'Bryant et al. 1988). To a point, there is an inverse dose–response relationship with injury prevention: The higher the neuromuscular training volume, the lower the risk of injury (Sugimoto et al. 2015; Sugimoto, Myer, Barber-Foss et al. 2014). In fact, program sessions lasting more than 30 minutes resulted in a 26 percent lower risk of ACL injury compared to programs performed for 15 minutes or less (Sugimoto, Myer, Barber-Foss et al. 2014). Thirty minutes per week is a relatively short amount of time and should be deemed the minimum for an injury prevention program (Sugimoto et al. 2015).

TABLE 11.5   ACL Injury Prevention Program: Intensity and Volume

	STRENGTH TRAINING EXERCISES	PLYOMETRIC TRAINING EXERCISES	SPECIAL TRAINING EXERCISES
PRESEASON	4 exercises	2 exercises	2 exercises
	2 sets of 8 each	2 sets of 10 each	2 sets of 10 each
IN-SEASON	3 exercises	2 exercises	2 exercises
	1 set of 6 each	1 set of 10 each	2 sets of 10 each
OFF-SEASON	6 exercises	4 exercises	None
	2 sets of 10 each	2-3 sets of 10 each	

SAMPLE PROGRAMS

In the sections that follow, we offer two sample injury prevention programs. One is focused on a specific sport (soccer; see tables 11.6-11.8) and the other is focused on a specific structure (hamstring; see tables 11.9-11.11). When reviewing these sample programs, note that the same format is used for each. Both an intermediate program and an advanced program are shown; there is overlap between them, but there are unique features for each as well. When designing injury prevention programs, follow the steps outlined in this chapter to make your programs specific to the needs of the teams, athletes, and anatomical structures they are intended to protect.

Soccer Injury Prevention

This soccer injury prevention program is an intermediate-level program and includes strength training, plyometric training, and special training exercises, which follow a warm-up. This program may be performed at any time during the year; the real change is the volume and frequency of the program.

TABLE 11.6   Soccer Injury Prevention Program: Warm-Up

EXERCISE	SETS	REPS/DISTANCE	PAGE
Walking lunge	1	10	189
Inverted hamstring stretch	1	10	190
Single-leg squat (with eyes closed)	1	10	112
Ankle flip	2	100 feet (30 m)	193
Single-leg stair bound	2	6	191
Shuffle	2	100 feet (30 m)	192
Pogo	2	10	166
Sprinting (50% effort)	6	100 feet (30 m)	N/A

TABLE 11.7   Soccer Injury Prevention Program: Day 1

EXERCISE TYPE	EXERCISE	SETS	REPS	LOAD	PAGE
PLYOMETRIC EXERCISES	Drop (depth) jump	2	10	18 inches (45 cm)	143
	Standing long jump to vertical jump	2	10	BWT*	151
	Single-leg vertical jump	2	10	BWT	145
	Standing long jump to single-leg landing	2	10	BWT	150
STRENGTH EXERCISES	Back squat	3	8	50% BWT	110
	Side lunge	2	10		99
SPECIAL EXERCISES	Single-leg Romanian deadlift	3	8	25% BWT	121
	Manual eccentric hip abduction	2	10		94
	Side-lying hip abduction	2	15		92
	Heel raise	2	15		164

*BWT: Bodyweight exercise or a percentage of BWT (e.g., 50% BWT indicates you should use a weight equal to half of your bodyweight)

TABLE 11.8 Soccer Injury Prevention Program: Day 2

EXERCISE TYPE	EXERCISE	SETS	REPS	LOAD	PAGE
PLYOMETRIC EXERCISES	Drop (depth) jump to 90-degree turn	2	10	18 inches (45 cm)	144
	Single-leg side-to-side hop (for alignment)	1	10	BWT*	146
	Single-leg push-off	2	10	BWT	113
	Side hurdle jump	2	10	BWT	147
STRENGTH EXERCISES	Single-leg squat	2	10	4 lb	112
	Deadlift	2	8	50% BWT	72
SPECIAL EXERCISES	Stability ball hamstring curl + single-leg bench bridge compound set	3	10	BWT	138 and 97
	Side plank	2	10	BWT	74
	Nordic hamstring curl	2	10	BWT	117
	Cable hip flexion	2	10	Band	125
	Resistance band inversion (slow and fast)	2	15	Band	172
	Resistance band eversion (slow and fast)	2	15	Band	176

*BWT: Bodyweight exercise or a percentage of BWT (e.g., 50% BWT indicates you should use a weight equal to half of your bodyweight)

Hamstring Injury Prevention

This hamstring injury prevention program is an advanced-level program and includes plyometric, strength training, and special exercises, which follow a warm-up.

TABLE 11.9 Hamstring Injury Prevention Program: Warm-Up

EXERCISE	SETS	REPS/DISTANCE	PAGE
Walking lunge	1	10	189
Inverted hamstring stretch	1	10	190
Single-leg squat (with eyes closed)	1	10	112
Fast skip	2	100 feet (30 m)	169
Ankle flip	2	100 feet (30 m)	193
Shuffle	2	100 feet (30 m)	192
Pogo	2	10	166

TABLE 11.10   Hamstring Injury Prevention Program: Day 1

EXERCISE TYPE	EXERCISE	SETS	REPS	LOAD	PAGE
PLYOMETRIC EXERCISES	Drop freeze	2	10	24 inches (60 cm)	142
	Pike jump	2	10	BWT	122
	Front single-leg push-off	2	10	18 inches (45 cm)	114
	Plyometric reverse bench bridge	2	10	BWT	116
STRENGTH EXERCISES	Back squat	2	8	8RM	110
	Side lunge	2	10	BWT	99
SPECIAL EXERCISES	Romanian deadlift	2	10	25% BWT	120
	Stability ball hamstring curl + single-leg bench bridge compound set	2	10	BWT	138 and 97
	Heel raise	2	15	BWT	164
	Nordic hamstring curl	2	10	BWT	117

*BWT: Bodyweight exercise or a percentage of BWT (e.g., 50% BWT indicates you should use a weight equal to half of your bodyweight)

8RM is an eight repetition maximum that is the heaviest weight you can lift with maximum effort for eight repetitions

TABLE 11.11   Hamstring Injury Prevention Program: Day 2

EXERCISE TYPE	EXERCISE	SETS	REPS	LOAD	PAGE
PLYOMETRIC EXERCISES	Drop (depth) jump	2	10	18 inches (45 cm)	143
	Cycled split squat jump	2	10	BWT	101
	Sprinting	1	6	100 feet (30 m)	N/A
STRENGTH EXERCISES	Single-leg squat	2	10	10	112
	Deadlift	2	8	50% BWT	72
SPECIAL EXERCISES	Heel walk	2	60 ft	BWT	174
	Resistance band inversion with plantarflexion	2	15	Band	173
	Stability ball hamstring curl	3	10	BWT	138
	Heel raise	2	15	BWT	164

*BWT: Bodyweight exercise or a percentage of BWT (e.g., 50% BWT indicates you should use a weight equal to half of your bodyweight)

It is not possible to prevent all injuries. But with a careful reliance on the principles of injury prevention and an understanding of anatomy and common injuries covered in this book, it is possible to reduce your risk of injury. The examples provided in this chapter should serve as a general template for building your own injury prevention program. It is important that your injury prevention program be performed consistently throughout the sporting year along with your general training program, practices, and games.

EXERCISE FINDER

Note: The exercises in each chapter include an icon to describe the type of exercise mode – strength, plyometric, or special training (speed and agility, flexibility, and aerobic endurance) – that applies predominantly to that exercise; see page x for further explanation.

HEAD, NECK, AND SHOULDER

STRENGTH

Cervical isometric—flexion   25
  Cervical isometric—extension   27
  Cervical isometric—side bending   27
Push-up with plus   28
  Elevated push-up with plus   29
Dumbbell shoulder press   30
  Barbell shoulder press   31
Dumbbell row   32
  Barbell bent-over row   33
Farmer's carry   34
  Unstable farmer's carry   35
Prone horizontal abduction   36
  Prone horizontal abduction at 100 degrees   37
Scaption   38
External rotation at 90 degrees   40
  External rotation at 90 degrees—fast   41
D2 flexion with band   42

ELBOW, WRIST, AND HAND

STRENGTH

Overhead triceps extension   54
  Triceps kickback   55
Barbell biceps curl   56
  Alternate dumbbell biceps curl   57
Barbell wrist extension   58
  Standing dumbbell wrist extension   59
Barbell wrist flexion   60
  Wrist roller   61
Forearm supination and pronation   62
  Forearm supination and pronation with bat   63

SPINE AND TRUNK

STRENGTH

Deadlift   72
Side plank   74
  Side plank with hip abduction   75
Half-kneeling PNF chop   76
  PNF medicine ball chop   77
Standing PNF lift   78
Reverse hyperextension   80
  Medicine ball overhead toss   81

PLYOMETRIC

Medicine ball side toss   82
  Shuffle to side toss   83

(continued)

HIP

STRENGTH

Side-lying hip abduction   92
  Wall isometric hip abduction   93
Manual eccentric hip abduction   94
  Closed chain eccentric hip abduction   95
  Resisted side step   95
Bench bridge or hip thrust   96
  Single-leg bench bridge   97
Forward lunge   98
  Side lunge   99

PLYOMETRIC

Split squat jump   100
  Cycled split squat jump   101

THIGH

STRENGTH

Back squat   110
  Slant board squat   112
  Single-leg squat   112
Reverse bench bridge   115
  Plyometric reverse bench bridge   116
Nordic hamstring curl   117
  Harop curl   119
  Razor curl   119
Romanian deadlift   120
  Single-leg Romanian deadlift   121
Hip flexor hold   124
  Cable hip flexion   125
Copenhagen hold   126
  Copenhagen hold with leg lift   127

PLYOMETRIC

Single-leg push-off   113
  Front single-leg push-off   114
Pike jump   122

KNEE

STRENGTH

Single-leg squat   136
  Levitating lunge   137
Leg extension   152
  Kettlebell leg extension   153
  Nordic quadriceps exercise   153

PLYOMETRIC

Drop (depth) jump   143
  Drop (depth) jump to second box   144
  Drop (depth) jump to 90-degree turn   144
Single-leg vertical jump   145
  Single-leg vertical jump—continuous   146
  Single-leg side-to-side hop   146
Side hurdle jump   147
  Side hurdle jump—continuous   149
  Single-leg side hurdle jump   149
Standing long jump to single-leg landing   150
  Standing long jump to vertical jump   151

SPECIAL

Stability ball hamstring curl   138
  Seated leg curl   139
Deceleration   140
  Drop freeze   142
  Stability hop   142

LEG, ANKLE, AND FOOT

STRENGTH

Resistance band inversion 172

Resistance band inversion with plantar-flexion 173

Heel walk 174

Manual eccentric dorsiflexion 175

Resistance band eversion 176

Isometric eversion 177

PLYOMETRIC

Pogo 166

Single-leg pogo 167

Relevé hold 170

Relevé landing hold 171

SPECIAL

Heel raise 164

Single-leg heel raise 165

Seated heel raise 165

Skip 168

Fast skip 169

Backward skip 169

Side skip 169

Short foot 178

Arch lift 179

Barefoot walk 180

WARM-UP FOR INJURY PREVENTION

PLYOMETRIC

Ankle flip 193

SPECIAL

Walking lunge 189

Inverted hamstring stretch 190

Single-leg stair bound 191

Shuffle 192

REFERENCES

Al Attar WS, Soomro N, Pappas E, Sinclair PJ, Sanders RH.How effective are F-MARC injury prevention programs for soccer players? A systematic review and meta-analysis. *Sports Med.* 2016;46:205-217. doi:10.1007/s40279-015-0404-x

Al Attar WA, Soomro N, Sinclair PJ, Pappas E, Sanders RH. Effect of injury prevention programs that include the nordic hamstring exercise on hamstring injury rates in soccer players: A systematic review and meta-analysis. *Sports Med.* 2017;47(5):907-916. doi:10.1007/s40279-016-0638-2

Aranda Y, Munuera PV. Plantar fasciitis and its relationship with hallux limitus. *J Am Podiatr Med Assoc.* 2014 May;104(3):263-268. doi:10.7547/0003-0538-104.3.263

Archbold, P., and G. Mezzadri. Iliotibial band syndrome. *Surgery of the Knee* 2014; 127–130. doi:10.1007/978-1-4471-5631-4_12.

Ardern CL, Ekås GR, Grindem H, et al. Prevention, diagnosis and management of paediatric ACL injuries. *Br J Sports Med.* 2018;52(20):1297-1298. doi:10.1136/bjsports-2018-099493

Ardern CL, Taylor NF, Feller JA, Webster KE. Fifty-five per cent return to competitive sport following anterior cruciate ligament reconstruction surgery: An updated systematic review and meta-analysis including aspects of physical functioning and contextual factors. *Br J Sports Med.* 2014;48(21):1543-1552. doi:10.1136/bjsports-2013-093398

Asmussen E, Bonde-Petersen F, Jorgensen K. Mechano-elastic properties of human muscles at different temperatures. *Acta Physiol Scand.* 1976 Jan;96(1):83-93. doi:10.1111/j.1748-1716.1976.tb10173.x

Augustsson J. Documentation of strength training for research purposes after ACL reconstruction. *Knee Surg Sports Traumatol Arthrosc.* 2013 Aug;21(8):1849-1855.

Ayala F, López-Valenciano A, Gámez Martín JA, et al. A preventive model for hamstring injuries in professional soccer: Learning algorithms. *Int J Sports Med.* 2019 May;40(5):344-353.

Barengo NC, Meneses-Echávez JF, Ramírez-Vélez R, Cohen DD, Tovar G, Bautista JE. The impact of the FIFA 11+ training program on injury prevention in football players: a systematic review. *Int J Environ Res Public Health.* 2014;11:11986-12000. doi:10.3390/ijerph111111986

Bates NA, Ford KR, Myer GD, Hewett TE. Impact differences in ground reaction force and center of mass between the first and second landing phases of a drop vertical jump and their implications for injury risk assessment. *J Biomech.* 2013;46(7):1237-1241. doi:10.1016/j.jbiomech.2013.02.024

Bergh U, Ekblom B. Influence of muscle temperature on maximal muscle strength and power output in human skeletal muscles. *Acta Physiol Scand.* 1979 Sep;107(1):33-37. doi:10.1111/j.1748-1716.1979.tb06439.x

Bishop D. Warm up I: potential mechanisms and the effects of passive warm up on exercise performance. *Sports Med.* 2003;33(6):439-454. doi:10.2165/00007256-200333060-00005

Bourne MN, Duhig SJ, Timmins RG, et al. Impact of the Nordic hamstring and hip extension exercises on hamstring architecture and morphology: implications for injury prevention. *Br J Sports Med.* 2017;51:469-477.

Brooks JH, Fuller CW, Kemp SP, et al. Incidence, risk, and prevention of hamstring muscle injuries in professional rugby union. *Am J Sports Med.* 2006 Aug;34(8):1297-1306.

Butterfield TA, Herzog W. Quantification of muscle fiber strain during in vivo repetitive stretch-shortening cycles. *J Appl Physiol.* 2005;99:593-602.

Cameron KL, Thompson BS, Peck KY, Owens BD, Marshall SW, Svoboda SJ. Normative values for the KOOS and WOMAC in a young athletic population: History of knee ligament injury is associated with lower scores. *Am J Sports Med.* 2013;41(3):582-589. doi:10.1177/0363546512472330

Cherni Y, Jlid MC, Mehrez H, et al. Eight Weeks of Plyometric Training Improves Ability to Change Direction and Dynamic Postural Control in Female Basketball Players. *Front Physiol.* 2019;10:726. Published 2019 Jun 13. doi:10.3389/fphys.2019.00726

Collins JD, Almonroeder TG, Ebersole KT, O'Connor KM. The effects of fatigue and anticipation on the mechanics of the knee during cutting in female athletes. *Clin Biomech* (Bristol, Avon). 2016;35:62-67. doi:10.1016/j.clinbiomech.2016.04.004

Crossley KM, Patterson BE, Culvenor AG, Bruder AM, Mosler AB, Mentiplay BF Making football safer for women: a systematic review and meta-analysis of injury prevention programmes in 11 773 female football (soccer) players. *Br J Sports Med.* 2020 Sep;54(18):1089-1098.

Darrall-Jones J, Roe G, Cremen E, Jones, B. Can team-sport athletes accurately run at submaximal sprinting speeds? implications for rehabilitation and warm-up protocols. *J Strength Cond Res.* 2021 Jan. doi:10.1519/JSC.0000000000003960

de Jonge S, van den Berg C, de Vos RJ, van der Heide HL, Weir A, Verhaar JN, Bierma-Zeinstra SA, Tol, JL. Incidence of midportion Achilles tendinopathy in the general population. *Br J Sports Med.* 2011;45(13):1026-1028.

Dello Iacono A, Vigotsky A, Laver L, Halperin I. Beneficial effects of small-sided games as a conclusive part of warm-up routines in young elite handball players. *J Strength Cond Res.* 2021 Jun;35(6):1724-1731. doi:10.1519/JSC.0000000000002983

deVries HA, Housh TJ. *Physiology of exercise for physical education, athletics and exercise science.* 5th ed. Brown; 1995.

Dickin DC, Johann E, Wang H, Popp JK. Combined effects of drop height and fatigue on landing mechanics in active females. *J Appl Biomech.* 2015;31(4):237-243. doi:10.1123/jab.2014-0190

Dix C, Logerstedt D, Arundale A, Snyder-Mackler L. Perceived barriers to implementation of injury prevention programs among collegiate women's soccer coaches. *J Sci Med Sport.* 2021 Apr;24(4):352-356. doi:10.1016/j.jsams.2020.09.016

Draghi F, Bortolotto C, Ferrozzi G. Soleus strain: an underestimated injury? [published online ahead of print, 2021 Jan 5]. *J Ultrasound.* doi:10.1007/s40477-020-00555-7

Drezner J, Ulager J, Sennett MD. Hamstring muscle injuries in track and field athletes: A 3-year study at the Penn Relay Carnival [abstract]. *Clin J Sport Med.* 2005;15(5):386.

Ekstrand J, Hägglund M, Waldén M. Injury incidence and injury patterns in professional football - the UEFA injury study [published online ahead of print, 2010 May 29. *Br J Sports Med.*

Enoka, RM. *Neuromechanics of Human Movement.* 5th ed. Human Kinetics; 2015.

Fairclough J, Hayashi K, Toumi H, et al. Is iliotibial band syndrome really a friction syndrome?. *J Sci Med Sport.* 2007;10(2):74-78. doi:10.1016/j.jsams.2006.05.017

Feeley BT, Kennelly S, Barnes RP, et al. Epidemiology of National Football League training camp injuries from 1998 to 2007. *Am J Sports Med.* 2008 Aug;36(8):1597-1603.

Fernandez-Fernandez J, García-Tormo V, Santos-Rosa FJ, et al. The effect of a neuromuscular vs. dynamic warm-up on physical performance in young tennis players. *J Strength Cond Res.* 2020 Oct;34(10):2776-2784. doi:10.1519/JSC.0000000000003703

Finch CF, Twomey DM, Fortington LV, et al. Preventing Australian football injuries with a targeted neuromuscular control exercise programme: comparative injury rates from a training intervention delivered in a clustered randomised controlled trial. *Inj Prev.* 2016 Apr;22(2):123-128.

Fleck S, Kraemer W. *Designing Resistance Training Programs.* 4th ed. Human Kinetics; 2014:1-62, 179-296.

Fong DT, Hong Y, Chan LK, Yung PS, Chan KM. A systematic review on ankle injury and ankle sprain in sports. *Sports Med.* 2007;37(1):73-94. doi:10.2165/00007256-200737010-00006

Ford K, Myer G, Schmitt L, van den Bogert A, Hewett, T. Effect of drop height on lower extremity biomechanical measures in female athletes. *Med Sci Sports Exerc.* 2008;40:S80.

Fradkin AJ, Gabbe BJ, Cameron PA. Does warming up prevent injury in sport? the evidence from randomised controlled trials? *J Sci Med Sport.* 2006 Jun;9(3):214-220. doi:10.1016/j.jsams.2006.03.026

Fradkin AJ, Zazryn TR, Smoliga JM. Effects of warming-up on physical performance: a systematic review with meta-analysis. *J Strength Cond Res.* 2010 Jan;24(1):140-148. doi:10.1519/JSC.0b013e3181c643a0

Frank BS, Gilsdorf CM, Goerger BM, Prentice WE, Padua DA. Neuromuscular fatigue alters postural control and sagittal plane hip biomechanics in active females with anterior cruciate ligament reconstruction. *Sports Health.* 2014;6(4):301-308. doi:10.1177/1941738114530950

Freckleton G, Cook J, Pizzari T. The predictive validity of a single leg bridge test for hamstring injuries in Australian Rules football players. *Br J Sports Med.* 2014;48:713-717.

Fuller M, Moyle GM, Minett GM. Injuries across a pre-professional ballet and contemporary dance tertiary training program: A retrospective cohort study. *J Sci Med Sport.* 2020;23(12):1166-1171. doi:10.1016/j.jsams.2020.06.012

Gabbett TJ, Hulin B, Blanch P, Chapman P, Bailey D. To couple or not to couple? For acute:chronic workload ratios and injury risk, does it really matter? *Int J Sports Med.* 2019;40(9):597-600. doi:10.1055/a-0955-5589

Gil MH, Neiva HP, Alves AR, et al. The effect of warm-up running technique on sprint performance [published online ahead of print, 2020 Mar 12]. *J Strength Cond Res.* doi:10.1519/JSC.0000000000003528

Gilchrist, J, Mandelbaum BR, Melancon H, et al. A randomized controlled trial to prevent noncontact anterior cruciate ligament injury in female collegiate soccer players. *Am J Sports Med.* 2008;36:1476-1483.

Goel R, Abzug JM. de Quervain's tenosynovitis: a review of the rehabilitative options. *Hand* (N Y). 2015 Mar;10(1):1-5.

Goodwill AM, Pearce AJ, Kidgell DJ. Corticomotor plasticity following unilateral strength training. *Muscle Nerve.* 2012 Sep;46(3):384-393.

Goossens L, Witvrouw E, Vanden Bossche L, et al. Lower eccentric hamstring strength and single leg hop for distance predict hamstring injury in PETE students. *Eur J Sport Sci* 2015;15:436-442.

Green B, Bourne MN, van Dyk N, Pizzari T. Recalibrating the risk of hamstring strain injury (HSI): A 2020 systematic review and meta-analysis of risk factors for index and recurrent hamstring strain injury in sport. *Br J Sports Med.* 2020;54(18):1081-1088. doi:10.1136/bjsports-2019-100983

Gremion G. Les exercices d'étirement dans la pratique sportive ont-ils encore leur raison d'être? Une revue de la littérature [Is stretching for sports performance still useful? A review of the literature]. *Rev Med Suisse.* 2005;1(28):1830-1834.

Grindstaff TL, Potach, DH. Prevention of common wrestling injuries. *Strength Cond J.* 2006 Aug;28(4):20-28.

Harwin JR, Richardson ML. "Tennis leg": gastrocnemius injury is a far more common cause than plantaris rupture. *Radiol Case Rep.* 2016;12(1):120-123. doi:10.1016/j.radcr.2016.10.012

Heiser TM, Weber J, Sullivan G, et al. Prophylaxis and management of hamstring muscle injuries in intercollegiate football players. *Am J Sports Med.* 1984 Sep-Oct;12(5):368-370.

Herman K, Barton C, Malliaras P, Morrissey D. The effectiveness of neuromuscular warm-up strategies, that require no additional equipment, for preventing lower limb injuries during sports participation: a systematic review. *BMC Med.* 2012;10:75. Published 2012 Jul 19. doi:10.1186/1741-7015-10-75

Hewett TE, Myer GD, Ford KR, et al. Biomechanical measures of neuromuscular control and valgus loading of the knee predict anterior cruciate ligament injury risk in female athletes: a prospective study. *Am J Sports Med.* 2005;33(4):492-501. doi:10.1177/0363546504269591

Hewett TE, Ford KR, Myer GD. Anterior cruciate ligament injuries in female athletes: Part 2, a meta-analysis of neuromuscular interventions aimed at injury prevention. *Am J Sports Med.* 2006;34(3):490-498. doi:10.1177/0363546505282619

Higashihara A, Nagano Y, Ono T, et al. Differences in hamstring activation characteristics between the acceleration and maximum-speed phases of sprinting. *J Sports Sci.* 2018;36:1313-1318.

Hiller CE, Nightingale EJ, Raymond J, et al. Prevalence and impact of chronic musculoskeletal ankle disorders in the community. *Arch Phys Med Rehabil.* 2012;93(10):1801-1807. doi:10.1016/j.apmr.2012.04.023

Hoffman J. *Physiological Aspects of Sport Training and Performance.* Human Kinetics; 2002.

Huang YL, Jung J, Mulligan CMS, Oh J, Norcross MF. A majority of anterior cruciate ligament injuries can be Prevented by injury prevention programs: a systematic review of randomized controlled trials and cluster-randomized controlled trials with meta-analysis. *Am J Sports Med.* 2020 May;48(6):1505-1515. doi:10.1177/0363546519870175

Hutchinson LA, Lichtwark GA, Willy RW, Kelly LA. The iliotibial band: A complex structure with versatile functions [published online ahead of print, 2022 Jan 24]. *Sports Med.* 2022;10.1007/s40279-021-01634-3. doi:10.1007/s40279-021-01634-3

Johansson F, Cools A, Gabbett T, Fernandez-Fernandez J, Skillgate E. Association between spikes in external training load and shoulder injuries in competitive adolescent tennis players: The SMASH cohort study. *Sports Health.* 2022;14(1):103-110. doi:10.1177/19417381211051643

Jones RI, Ryan B, Todd AI. Muscle fatigue induced by a soccer match-play simulation in amateur Black South African players. *J Sports Sci.* 2015;33(12):1305-1311. doi:10.1080/02640414.2015.1022572

Khayambashi K, Ghoddosi N, Straub RK, Powers CM. Hip muscle strength predicts noncontact anterior cruciate ligament injury in male and female athletes: a prospective study. *Am J Sports Med.* 2016 Feb;44(2):355-361.

Klugman MF, Brent JL, Myer GD, Ford KR, Hewett TE. Does an in-season only neuromuscular training protocol reduce deficits quantified by the tuck jump assessment? *Clin Sports Med.* 2011;30:825-840.

Knapik JJ, Bauman CL, Jones BH, Harris JM, Vaughan L. Preseason strength and flexibility imbalances associated with athletic injuries in female collegiate athletes. *Am J Sports Med.* 1991;19:76-81.

Kongsgaard M, Aagaard P, Roikjaer S, Olsen D, Jensen M, Langberg H. Decline eccentric squats increases patellar tendon loading compared to standard eccentric squats. *Clin Biomech* (Bristol, Avon). 2006;21:748-754.

Kumagai K, Abe T, Brechue WF, Ryushi T, Takano S, Mizuno M. Sprint performance is related to muscle fascicle length in male 100-m sprinters. *J Appl Physiol* (1985). 2000;88(3):811-816. doi:10.1152/jappl.2000.88.3.811

Landorf KB, Kaminski MR, Munteanu SE, Zammit GV, Menz HB. Clinical measures of foot posture and ankle joint dorsiflexion do not differ in adults with and without plantar heel pain. *Sci Rep.* 2021 Mar 19;11(1):6451. doi:10.1038/s41598-021-85520-y

Markolf KL, Burchfield DM, Shapiro MM, Shepard MF, Finerman GA, Slauterbeck JL. Combined knee loading states that generate high anterior cruciate ligament forces. *J Orthop Res.* 1995;13(6):930-935. doi:10.1002/jor.1100130618

Martinez JC, Mazerolle SM, Denegar CR, et al. Female adolescent athletes' attitudes and perspectives on injury prevention programs. *J Sci Med Sport.* 2017;20(2):146-151. doi:10.1016/j.jsams.2016.06.009

Marušič J, Vatovec R, Markovič G, Šarabon N. Effects of eccentric training at long-muscle length on architectural and functional characteristics of the hamstrings. *Scand J Med Sci Sports.* 2020 Nov;30(11):2130-2142.

Mawson R, Creech MJ, Peterson DC et al. Lower limb injury prevention programs in youth soccer: a survey of coach knowledge, usage, and barriers. *J Exp Orthop.* 2018;5:43. doi:10.1186/s40634-018-0160-6

Mayo M, Seijas R, Alvarez P. Structured neuromuscular warm-up for injury prevention in young elite football players. *Rev Esp Cir Ortop Traumatol.* 2014;58:336-342. doi:10.1016/j.recote.2014.09.004

McArdle WD, Katch FI, Katch VL. *Exercise Physiology: Nutrition, Energy, and Human Performance.* 8th ed. LWW; 2014.

McBride JM, McCaulley GO, Cormie P, Nuzzo JL, Cavill MJ, Triplett NT. Comparison of methods to quantify volume during resistance exercise. *J Strength Cond Res.* 2009 Jan;23(1):106-110.

McGowan CJ, Pyne DB, Thompson KG, Rattray B. Warm-up strategies for sport and exercise: Mechanisms and applications. *Sports Med.* 2015;45:1523-1546.

Mendiguchia J, Conceição F, Edouard P, et al. Sprint versus isolated eccentric training: comparative effects on hamstring architecture and performance in soccer players. *PLoS One.* 2020 Feb 11;15(2):e0228283. doi:10.1371/journal.pone.0228283

Miranda DL, Fadale PD, Hulstyn MJ, Shalvoy RM, Machan JT, Fleming BC. Knee biomechanics during a jump-cut maneuver: effects of sex and ACL surgery. *Med Sci Sports Exerc.* 2013 May;45(5):942-951.

Moffroid MT, Haugh LD, Haig AJ, Henry SM, Pope MH. Endurance training of trunk extensor muscles. *Phys Ther.* 1993;73:10-17.

Moore D, Semciw AI, Pizzari T. A systematic review and meta-analysis of common therapeutic exercises that generate highest muscle activity in the gluteus medius and gluteus minimus segments. *Int J Sports Phys Ther.* 2020;15(6):856-881. doi:10.26603/ijspt20200856

Morin JB, Gimenez P, Edouard P, et al. Sprint acceleration mechanics: the major role of hamstrings in horizontal force production. *Front Physiol.* 2015;6:404. doi:10.3389/fphys.2015.00404

Myer GD, Brent JL, Ford KR, Hewett TE.. A pilot study to determine the effect of trunk and hip focused neuromuscular training on hip and knee isokinetic strength. *Br J Sports Med.* 2008;42:614-619.

Myer GD, Faigenbaum AD, Foss KB, et al. Injury initiates unfavourable weight gain and obesity markers in youth. *Br J Sports Med.* 2013;48(20):1477-1481. doi:10.1136/bjsports-2012-091988

Myer GD, Ford KR, Barber Foss KD, Liu C, Nick TG, Hewett TE. The relationship of hamstrings and quadriceps strength to anterior cruciate ligament injury in female athletes. *Clin J Sport Med.* 2009 Jan;19(1):3-8.

Myer GD, Ford KR, Brent JL, Hewett TE. Differential neuromuscular training effects on ACL injury risk factors in "high-risk" versus "low-risk" athletes. *BMC musculoskeletal disorders.* 2007;8:39.

Myer GD, Ford KR, Brent JL, Hewett TE. The effects of plyometric versus dynamic balance training on power, balance and landing force in female athletes. *J Strength Cond Res.* 2006;20:345-353.

Myer GD, Ford KR, Hewett TE. Rationale and clinical techniques for anterior cruciate ligament injury prevention among female athletes. *J Athl Train*. 2004;39:352-364.

Myer GD, Ford KR, Khoury J, Succop P, Hewett TE. Biomechanics laboratory-based prediction algorithm to identify female athletes with high knee loads that increase risk of ACL injury. *Br J Sports Med*. 2011 Apr;45(4):245-252.

Myer GD, Ford KR, McLean SG, Hewett TE. The effects of plyometric versus dynamic stabilization and balance training on lower extremity biomechanics. *Am J Sports Med*. 2006;34:445-455.

Myer GD, Ford KR, Palumbo JP, Hewett TE. Neuromuscular training improves performance and lower-extremity biomechanics in female athletes. *J Strength Cond Res*. 2005;19:51-60.

Myer GD, Lloyd RS, Brent JL, Faigenbaum AD. How young is "too young" to start training? *ACSMs Health Fit J*. 2013;17:14-23.

Myer GD, Stroube BW, DiCesare CA, et al. Augmented feedback supports skill transfer and reduces high-risk injury landing mechanics: a double-blind, randomized controlled laboratory study. *Am J Sports Med*. 2013;41:669-677.

National Strength and Conditioning Association, Haff G, Travis TN. *Essentials of strength training and conditioning*. 4th ed. Human Kinetics; 2016:440.

Niederbracht Y, Shim AL, Sloniger MA, Paternostro-Bayles M, Short TH. Effects of a shoulder injury prevention strength training program on eccentric external rotator muscle strength and glenohumeral joint imbalance in female overhead activity athletes. *J Strength Cond Res*. 2008 Jan;22(1):140-145.

Noyes FR, Barber Westin SD. Anterior cruciate ligament injury prevention training in female athletes: a systematic review of injury reduction and results of athletic performance tests. *Sports Health*. 2012 Jan;4(1):36-46. doi:10.1177/1941738111430203

Nussbaum ED, Hosea TM, Sieler SD, Incremona BR, Kessler DE. Prospective evaluation of syndesmotic ankle sprains without diastasis. *Am J Sports Med*. 2001;29:31-35.

O'Bryant HS, Byrd R, Stone MH. Cycle ergometer performance and maximum leg and hip strength adaptations to two different methods of weight-training. *J Strength Conditioning Res*. 1988;2(2):27-30.

O'Connor KM, Johnson C, Benson LC. The effect of isolated hamstrings fatigue on landing and cutting mechanics. *J Appl Biomech*. 2015;31(4):211-220. doi:10.1123/jab.2014-0098

Okoroha KR, Conte S, Makhni EC, et al. Hamstring injury trends in Major and Minor League Baseball: epidemiological findings from the Major League Baseball health and injury tracking system. *Orthop J Sports Med*. 2019;7(7):2325967119861064. doi:10.1177/2325967119861064

Olewnik L, Wysiadecki G, Polguj M, Topol M. The report on the co-occurrence of two different rare anatomic variations of the plantaris muscle tendon on both sides of an individual. *Folia Morphologica* (Poland). 2017;76(2):331-333.

Oliveira FB, Oliveira AS, Rizatto GF, Denadai BS. Resistance training for explosive and maximal strength: effects on early and late rate of force development. *J Sports Sci Med*. 2013 Sep 1;12(3):402-408.

Oliver GD, Dougherty CP. The razor curl: a functional approach to hamstring training. *J Strength Cond Res.* 2009 Mar;23(2):401-405. doi:10.1519/JSC.0b013e31818f08d0

Opplert J, Babault N. Acute effects of dynamic stretching on muscle flexibility and performance: An analysis of the current literature. *Sports Med.* 2018;48(2):299-325. doi:10.1007/s40279-017-0797-9

Palmieri-Smith RM, McLean SG, Ashton-Miller JA, Wojtys EM. Association of quadriceps and hamstrings cocontraction patterns with knee joint loading. *J Athl Train.* 2009;44(3):256-263. doi:10.4085/1062-6050-44.3.256

Paterno MV, Rauh MJ, Schmitt LC, Ford KR, Hewett TE. Incidence of second ACL injuries 2 years after primary ACL reconstruction and return to sport. *Am J Sports Med.* 2014;42(7):1567-1573. PMCID: PMC4205204

Paterno MV, Schmitt LC, Ford KR, et al. *Am J Sports Med.* 2010 Oct;38(10):1968-1978.

Petushek EJ, Sugimoto D, Stoolmiller M, Smith G, Myer GD. Evidence-based best-practice guidelines for preventing anterior cruciate ligament injuries in young female athletes: a systematic review and meta-analysis. *Am J Sports Med.* 2019 Jun;47(7):1744-1753.

Pollard CD, Sigward SM, Powers CM. ACL injury prevention training results in modification of hip and knee mechanics during a drop-landing task. *Orthop J Sports Med.* 2017 Sep 8;5(9):2325967117726267. doi:10.1177/2325967117726267

Potach DH, Myer G, Grindstaff, TL. Special consideration: female athlete and ACL injury prevention. In: Parikh SN, editor. *The Pediatric Anterior Cruciate Ligament.* Springer; 2018:251-283.

Powell RW. Lawn tennis leg. *Lancet.* 1883;122(3123):44.

Prince C, Morin JB, Mendiguchia J, et al. Sprint specificity of isolated hamstring-strengthening exercises in terms of muscle activity and force production. *Front Sports Act Living.* 2021 Jan 21;2:609636. doi:10.3389/fspor.2020.609636

Proske U, Morgan DL. Muscle damage from eccentric exercise: mechanism, mechanical signs, adaptation and clinical applications. *J Physiol.* 2001;537:333-345.

Quatman CE, Hewett TE. The anterior cruciate ligament injury controversy: is "valgus collapse" a sex-specific mechanism? *Br J Sports Med.* 2009;43:328-335.

Rodríguez C, Echegoyen S, Aoyama T. The effects of "Prevent injury and Enhance Performance Program" in a female soccer team. *J Sports Med Phys Fitness.* 2018 May;58(5):659-663. doi:10.23736/S0022-4707.17.07024-4

Rössler R, Verhagen E, Rommers N, et al. Comparison of the "11+ Kids" injury prevention programme and a regular warmup in children's football (soccer): a cost effectiveness analysis. *Br J Sports Med.* 2019 Mar;53(5):309-314. doi:10.1136/bjsports-2018-099395

Sá MA, Neto GR, Costa PB, et al. Acute effects of different stretching techniques on the number of repetitions in a single lower body resistance training session. *J Hum Kinet.* 2015;45:177-185. Published 2015 Apr 7. doi:10.1515/hukin-2015-0018

Sands WA. Injury prevention in women's gymnastics. *Sports Med.* 2000;30(5):359-373. doi:10.2165/00007256-200030050-00004

Schneider DK, Grandhi RK, Bansal P, et al. Current state of concussion prevention strategies: a systematic review and meta-analysis of prospective, controlled studies. *Br J Sports Med.* 2017 Oct;51(20):1473-1482.

Schuermans J, Van Tiggelan D, Danneels L, et al. Susceptibility to hamstring injuries in soccer: a prospective study using muscle functional magnetic resonance imaging. *Am J Sports Med.* 2016;44:1276-1285.

Sell TC, Ferris CM, Abt JP, et al. Predictors of proximal tibia anterior shear force during a vertical stop-jump. *J Orthop Res.* 2007;25(12):1589-1597.

Shiri R, Coggon D, Falah-Hassani K. Exercise for the prevention of low back pain: systematic review and meta-analysis of controlled trials. *Am J Epidemiol.* 2018 May;187(5):1093-1101.

Shrier I. Stretching before exercise: an evidence based approach. *Br J Sports Med.* 2000 Oct;34(5):324-325. doi:10.1136/bjsm.34.5.324

Shrier I. Stretching before exercise does not reduce the risk of local muscle injury: a critical review of the clinical and basic science literature. *Clin J Sport Med.* 1999 Oct;9(4):221-227. doi:10.1097/00042752-199910000-00007

Shultz SJ, Schmitz RJ, Cone JR, et al. Changes in fatigue, multiplanar knee laxity, and landing biomechanics during intermittent exercise. *J Athl Train.* 2015;50(5):486-497. doi:10.4085/1062-6050-49.5.08

Silva LM, Neiva HP, Marques MC, Izquierdo M, Marinho DA. Effects of warm-up, post-warm-up, and re-warm-up strategies on explosive efforts in team sports: A systematic review. *Sports Med.* 2018;48:2285-2299.

Silvers HJ, Mandelbaum BR. Preseason conditioning to prevent soccer injuries in young women. *Clin J Sport Med.* 2001 Jul;11(3):206.

Silvers-Granelli H, Mandelbaum B, Adeniji O, et al. Efficacy of the FIFA 11+ injury prevention program in the collegiate male soccer player. *Am J Sports Med.* 2015 Nov;43(11):2628-2637. doi:10.1177/0363546515602009

Söderman K, Alfredson H, Pietilä T, Werner S.. Risk factors for leg injuries in female soccer players: a prospective investigation during one out-door season. *Knee Surg Sports Traumatol Arthrosc.* 2001;9:313-321.

Stearns-Reider KM, Straub RK, Powers CM. Hip abductor rate of torque development as opposed to isometric strength predicts peak knee valgus during landing: implications for anterior cruciate ligament injury. *J Appl Biomech.* 2021 Sep 20;37(5):471-476.

Stone MH, Sands WA, Pierce KC, Ramsey MW, Haff GG. Power and power potentiation among strength-power athletes: preliminary study. *Int J Sports Physiol Perform.* 2008 Mar;3(1):55-67. doi:10.1123/ijspp.3.1.55

Stroube BW, Myer GD, Brent JL, Ford KR, Heidt RS, Jr., Hewett TE. Effects of task-specific augmented feedback on deficit modification during performance of the tuck-jump exercise. *J Sport Rehabil.* 2013;22:7-18.

Sugimoto D, Mattacola CG, Bush HM, et al. Preventive neuromuscular training for young female athletes: comparison of coach and athlete compliance rates. *J Athl Train.* 2017;52(1):58-64. doi:10.4085/1062-6050-51.12.20

Sugimoto D, Myer GD, Bush HM, Hewett TE. Effects of compliance on trunk and hip integrative neuromuscular training on hip abductor strength in female athletes. *J Strength Cond Res.* 2014;28:1187-1194.

Sugimoto D, Myer GD, Bush HM, Klugman MF, Medina McKeon JM, Hewett TE. Compliance with neuromuscular training and anterior cruciate ligament injury risk reduction in female athletes: a meta-analysis. *J Athl Train*. 2012;47:714-723.

Sugimoto D, Myer GD, Micheli LJ, Hewett TE. ABCs of evidence-based anterior cruciate ligament injury prevention strategies in female athletes. *Curr Phys Med Rehabil Rep*. 2015;3(1):43-49. doi:10.1007/s40141-014-0076-8

Sugimoto D, Myer G, Barber-Foss K, Hewett T. Dosage effects of neuromuscular training intervention to reduce anterior cruciate ligament injuries in female athletes: Meta- and sub-group analyses. *Sports Med*. 2014;44:551-562.

Swanson J. A functional approach to warm-up and flexibility. *Strength Cond J*. 2006;28:30-36.

Taddei UT, Matias AB, Duarte M, Sacco ICN. Foot core training to prevent running-related injuries: a survival analysis of a single-blind, randomized controlled trial. *Am J Sports Med*. 2020 Dec;48(14):3610-3619.

Takeuchi K, Takemura M, Nakamura M, Tsukuda F, Miyakawa S. Effects of active and passive warm-ups on range of motion, strength, and muscle passive properties in ankle plantarflexor muscles. *J Strength Cond Res*. 2021 Jan;35(1):141-146. doi:10.1519/JSC.0000000000002642

Tamura A, Akasaka K, Otsudo T, et al. Fatigue alters landing shock attenuation during a single-leg vertical drop jump. *Orthop J Sports Med*. 2016;4(1):2325967115626412. Published 2016 Jan 14. doi:10.1177/2325967115626412

Tanaka MJ, Jones LC, Forman JM. Awareness of anterior cruciate ligament injury: preventive training programs among female collegiate athletes. *J Athl Train*. 2020 Apr;55(4):359-364.

Tyler TF, Silvers HJ, Gerhardt MB, Nicholas SJ. Groin injuries in sports medicine. *Sports Health*. 2010;2(3):231-236. doi:10.1177/1941738110366820

van der Horst N, Smits DW, Petersen J, Goedhart EA, Backx FJ. The preventive effect of the Nordic hamstring exercise on hamstring injuries in amateur soccer players: study protocol for a randomised controlled trial. *Inj Prev*. 2014;20(4):e8. doi:10.1136/injuryprev-2013-041092

van Dyk N, Behan FP, Whiteley R. Including the Nordic hamstring exercise in injury prevention programmes halves the rate of hamstring injuries: a systematic review and meta-analysis of 8459 athletes. *Br J Sports Med*. 2019;53:1362-1370.

Vuurberg G, Hoorntje A, Wink LM, et al. Diagnosis, treatment and prevention of ankle sprains: update of an evidence-based clinical guideline. *Br J Sports Med*. 2018 Aug;52(15):956. doi:10.1136/bjsports-2017-098106

Warden SJ, Davis IS, Fredericson M. Management and prevention of bone stress injuries in long-distance runners. *J Orthop Sports Phys Ther*. 2014 Oct;44(10):749-765.

Webster KE, Hewett TE. Meta-analysis of meta-analyses of anterior cruciate ligament injury reduction training programs. *J Orthop Res*. 2018 Oct;36(10):2696-2708. doi:10.1002/jor.24043

Weier AT, Pearce AJ, Kidgell DJ. Strength training reduces intracortical inhibition. *Acta Physiol (Oxf)*. 2012 Oct;206(2):109-119.

Whittaker JL, Woodhouse LJ, Nettel-Aguirre A, Emery CA. Outcomes associated with early post-traumatic osteoarthritis and other negative health consequences 3-10 years following knee joint injury in youth sport. *Osteoarthritis Cartilage.* 2015;23(7):1122-1129. doi:10.1016/j.joca.2015.02.021

Wilk KE, Lupowitz LG, Arrigo CA. The youth throwers ten exercise program: A variation of an exercise series for enhanced dynamic shoulder control in the youth overhead throwing athlete. *Int J Sports Phys Ther.* 2021;16(6):1387-1395. Published 2021 Dec 1. doi:10.26603/001c.29923

Will JS, Bury DC, Miller JA. Mechanical low back pain. *Am Fam Physician.* 2018 Oct 1;98(7):421-428.

Withrow TJ, Huston LJ, Wojtys EM, Ashton-Miller JA. Effect of varying hamstring tension on anterior cruciate ligament strain during in vitro impulsive knee flexion and compression loading. *J Bone Joint Surg Am.* 2008;90:815-823.

Witvrouw E, Mahieu N, Danneels L, McNair P. Stretching and injury prevention: an obscure relationship. *Sports Med.* 2004;34(7):443-449. doi:10.2165/00007256-200434070-00003

Yamaguchi T, Ishii K, Yamanaka M, Yasuda K. Acute effect of static stretching on power output during concentric dynamic constant external resistance leg extension. *J Strength Cond Res.* 2006;20(4):804-810. doi:10.1519/R-18715.1

Young W, Behm D. Should static stretching be used during a warm-up for strength and power activities? *NSCA Journal.* 2002;24(6):33-37.

Yu B, Lin CF, Garrett WE. Lower extremity biomechanics during the landing of a stop-jump task. *Clin Biomech* (Bristol, Avon). 2006;21(3):297-305.

Zebis MK, Andersen LL, Bencke J, Kjaer M, Aagaard P. Identification of athletes at future risk of anterior cruciate ligament ruptures by neuromuscular screening. *Am J Sports Med.* 2009 Oct;37(10):1967-1973.

ADDITIONAL REFERENCE

International Olympic Committee Pediatric ACL Injury Consensus Group, Ardern CL, Ekås G, et al. 2018 International Olympic Committee consensus statement on prevention, diagnosis, and management of pediatric anterior cruciate ligament injuries. *Orthop J Sports Med.* 2018 Mar 21;6(3):2325967118759953.

ABOUT THE AUTHORS

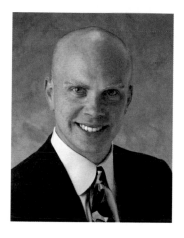

David Potach, PT, SCS, CSCS, is a director of physical rehabilitation at Cheshire Medical Center in Dartmouth, New Hampshire. He has been helping athletes reach their performance goals for over 20 years. Potach previously served as a strength and conditioning coach at Creighton University, was owner of Omaha Sports Physical Therapy, and was director of sports rehab at Children's Hospital and Medical Center.

Potach has spoken internationally and regionally on strength training and conditioning, plyometrics, injury prevention, and sports rehabilitation. He has authored several articles on sports rehabilitation as well as textbook chapters on sports medicine and sports conditioning. In 2005, he became one of the first recipients to be awarded the National Strength and Conditioning Association (NSCA) Sports Medicine/Rehabilitation Specialist of the Year award.

He is a board-certified sports physical therapist and is certified by the NSCA as a strength and conditioning specialist (CSCS) and personal trainer (NSCA-CPT). He holds master of physical therapy and master of science degrees—both from the University of Nebraska—and a bachelor of arts degree in exercise science from Creighton University.

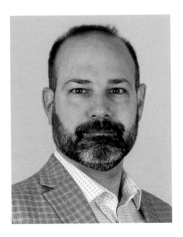

Erik P. Meira, PT, DPT, is currently the director of Physical Therapy Science Communication Group, a company based out of Portland, Oregon, that specializes in sports rehabilitation and education. He is also a clinical advisor to the University of Portland NCAA Division I program. He is an ABPTS board-certified sports clinical specialist and is certified by the NSCA as a strength and conditioning specialist (CSCS) with extensive experience in the management of sport injuries at many different levels. He is a frequent consultant for organizations within the NCAA, NBA, NFL, MLS, WNSL, and other elite sports leagues.

Dr. Meira has authored several articles and textbook chapters, and he lectures internationally, in settings that range from speaking to small teams in private settings to being the keynote speaker at large professional conferences. Known for his ability to make complex ideas simple to understand with a humorous delivery style, he covers topics such as hips, knees, exercise prescription, returning athletes to sport, science application, applied biomechanics, and physical therapy practice models. He was the founder and the original chair of the hip special interest group of the American Academy of Sports Physical Therapy (AASPT), served as their APTA Combined Sections Meeting (CSM) program chair, and was a member of the AASPT executive committee. He is also the cohost of PT Inquest, a podcast dedicated to understanding physical therapy science, and provides continuing education through The Science PT.

ANATOMY SERIES

Each book in the *Anatomy Series* provides detailed, full-color anatomical illustrations of the muscles in action and step-by-step instructions that detail perfect technique and form for each pose, exercise, movement, stretch, and stroke.

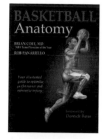

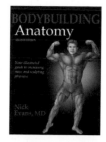

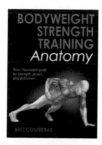

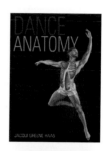

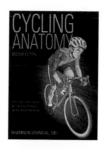

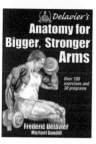

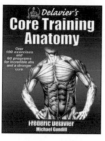

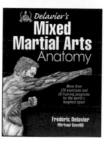

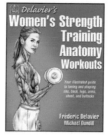

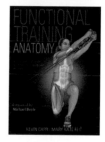

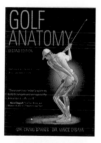

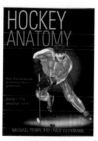

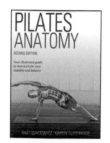

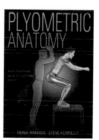

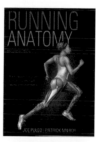

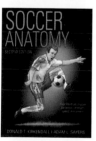

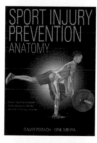

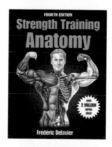

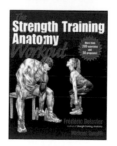

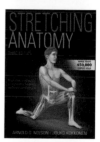

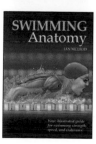

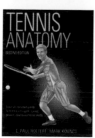

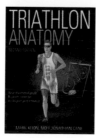

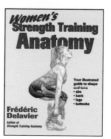

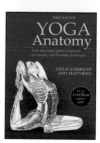

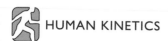

HUMAN KINETICS

U.S. 1-800-747-4457 • US.HumanKinetics.com/collections/anatomy
Canada 1-800-465-7301 • Canada.HumanKinetics.com/collections/anatomy
International 1-217-351-5076

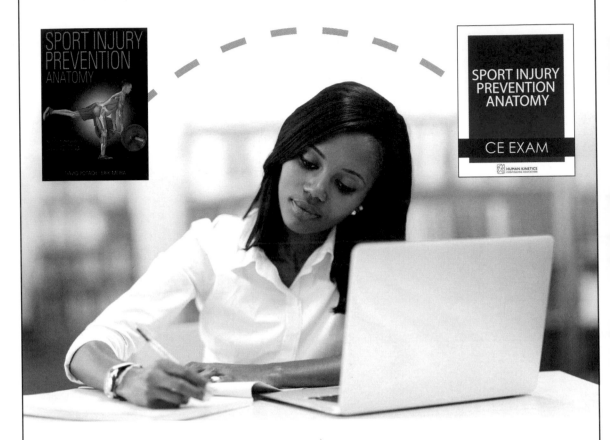
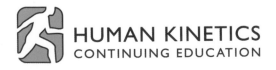